MEDICAL OFFICE
PHARMACOLOGY

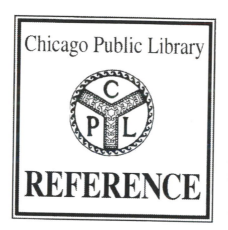

MEDICAL OFFICE PHARMACOLOGY

Barb R. Struck, RHIT
Lake Superior College
Duluth, Minnesota

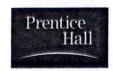

Prentice Hall
Upper Saddle River, New Jersey 07458

Library of Congress Cataloging-in-Publication Data

Struck, Barb R.
    Medical office pharmacology / Barb R. Struck
      p. cm.
    Includes bibliographical references and index.
    ISBN 0-8359-5290-8
    1. Pharmacology. 2. Medical assistants. I. Title.
    [DNLM: 1. Pharmacology. 2. Drug Therapy—
  methods. 3. Pharmaceutical Preparations—
  administration & dosage. QV 4 S927m 2000]
  RM301 .S75 2000
  615′.1—dc21

                          00-029859

Publisher: Julie Alexander
Acquisitions Editor: Barbara Krawiec
Director of Production
  and Manufacturing: Bruce Johnson
Managing Production Editor: Patrick Walsh
Production Editor: Kristen Butler, BookMasters, Inc.
Production Liaison: Danielle Newhouse
Senior Production Manager: Ilene Sanford
Creative Director: Marianne Frasco
Cover Design Coordinator: Maria Guglielmo
Director of Marketing: Leslie Cavaliere
Marketing Coordinator: Cindy Frederick
Editorial Assistant: Melissa Kerian
Composition: BookMasters, Inc.
Printing and Binding: The Banta Company

Prentice-Hall International (UK) Limited, *London*
Prentice-Hall of Australia Pty. Limited, *Sydney*
Prentice-Hall Canada Inc., *Toronto*
Prentice-Hall Hispanoamericana, S.A., *Mexico*
Prentice-Hall of India Private Limited, *New Delhi*
Prentice-Hall of Japan, Inc., *Tokyo*
Prentice-Hall Singapore Pte. Ltd.
Editora Prentice-Hall do Brasil, Ltda., *Rio de Janeiro*

Notice: The author and the publisher of this book have taken care to make certain that the equipment, doses of drugs and schedules of treatment are correct and compatible with the standards generally accepted at the time of publication. Nevertheless, as new information becomes available, changes in treatment and in the use of equipment and drugs become necessary. The reader is advised to carefully consult the instruction and information material included in the package insert of each drug or therapeutic agent, piece of equipment or device before administration. This advice is especially important when using new or infrequently used drugs. Health care workers are warned that use of any drugs or techniques must be authorized by their medical advisor, in accord with local laws and regulations. The publisher disclaims any liability, loss, injury, or damage incurred as a consequence, directly or indirectly, of the use and application of any of the contents of this book.

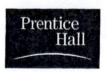

10 9 8 7 6 5 4 3 2
ISBN 0-8359-5290-8

Brief Contents

APPENDICES

Contents

Chapter 3. Drug Sources and Forms   21

Chapter 4. Drug Dosages and Effects   32

Chapter 5. Routes, Methods, and Documentation of Medication Administration   43

APPENDICES

Preface

This text comes to you with much pride, excitement, and satisfaction! Each chapter in this book was written, reviewed, rewritten, re-reviewed, for the majority of the last 4 years. Without the commitment of my pharmacist consultant and the reviewers who provided their knowledge, experience, and expertise, this text could not have been published. Every critique was invaluable and every comment, positive as well as negative, was appreciated. I am truly grateful for the assistance I received.

Medical Office Pharmacology was designed specifically for use in secretarial teaching facilities, vocational/technical schools, and community colleges, and is intended for use in the following programs: Medical Receptionist, Medical Secretary (both diploma and degree), Medical Transcription, and Medical Diagnostic Coding. Because it is designed as an entry-level text, it is also appropriate for first semester Medical Assistant students. It can be used as a stand-alone text or incorporated as a supplement with other required textbooks. To maximize student learning, the text should be used in conjunction with or following a medical terminology course.

Key Features:

- **Easy readability** to meet the learning needs of all students.
- **Learning objectives** are clearly listed at the beginning of each chapter. These objectives address the concepts the learner should understand and allow immediate feedback on progress.
- **Practice exercises** challenge the learner's knowledge and application of the material presented. The review exercises at the end of the chapters focus on main objectives and reinforce the most important points in the chapter. There are a wide variety of exercises ranging from multiple choice, short answer, matching, true/false, and fill-in-the-blanks.
- **Comprehensive appendices** for quick reference of commonly used abbreviations and symbols, medical terminology elements, commonly prescribed drugs, and look-alike sound-alike drugs.

- A **comprehensive Instructor's Manual** includes chapter objectives, a sample syllabus, a sample final exam with answers, and provides answers to the students' review questions.

ACKNOWLEDGMENTS

I wish to express my deepest gratitude to the people who so willingly offered enthusiasm, encouragement, optimism, reassurance, and advice as I worked diligently on completing this book.

My deepest thanks are due especially to the following people who acted as consultants and assisted in reviewing various parts of the manuscript. Without their expertise, comments, suggestions, and recommendations, this book would not have been possible. Again, each and every critique was invaluable and I appreciate every comment, positive as well as negative. I am truly grateful for your assistance.

I extend my gratitude to my consultant pharmacist, Craig Witchall, RPh; Medical Arts Pharmacy; Duluth, Minnesota; whom I called on *numerous* occasions for help.

Reviewers:

Marie A. Moisio, MA, RRA
Medical Secretary Program
Northern Michigan University
Marquette, MI

Kate McNally
Coordinator
Continuing Education
Des Moines Area Community College
Ankeny, IA

Karon K. Stejskal
Medical Secretary Instructor
Itasca Community College
Grand Rapids, MN

Patricia W. Burns
Professor
Business/Office Technology (Retired)

Jean Ure
Medical Office Technology Instructor
Rolla Technical Institute
Rolla, MO

Dr. K. Minchella, CMA
Medical Consultant
Past President of the Michigan Society of Medical Assistants
Liaison with American Academy of Family Physicians

My coworkers from Lake Superior College in Duluth, MN who, for 4 years, helped me solve word-processing problems and listened to me cry, brag, and complain on almost a daily basis:

Linda Grayson	June Siiter
Janet Gabel	Tina Johnson
Karen Pearson	Joyce Nelson
Nancy Swanson	

Friends who provided their expertise and encouragement for me to follow through on this endeavor:

Randy Visconi

Dennis Nelson

To the 4 years of students who bore with me as I used them to "try out" new material.

And last but not least, I express my gratitude and heartfelt thanks for the encouragement of my family, who on a weekly basis for these 4 years would subtly ask "and how is *the book* coming?":

Bob, Seth, Alex, Mom, Dad, Diane, and Deb.

Thank you and I love you!

MEDICAL OFFICE
PHARMACOLOGY

Introduction to Pharmacology

This chapter briefly covers the evolution of medicine and pharmacology. There have been substantial developments and advances in the health care field in recent years. Although the medical assistant, medical transcriptionist, coder, and medical secretary do *not* prescribe medication, they will be indirectly working with drugs on a daily basis. Individuals take medicine for various reasons; this chapter reviews the reasons medications are prescribed.

PHARMACOLOGY

Pharmacology, the science that deals with the study of chemical substances and their effects on living organisms, is one of the oldest branches of medicine. It is also concerned with the history, sources, and physical properties of drugs.

There are several subdivisions of pharmacology. Four of these subdivisions are listed as follows.

1. **Pharmacodynamics** is the study of drugs and their actions on the body;
2. **Pharmacokinetics** is the study of the metabolism and action of drugs within the body with particular emphasis on the time required for absorption, duration, distribution, and method of excretion;
3. **Pharmacotherapeutics** studies the relationship between drugs and the treatment of diseases; and
4. **Toxicology** is the study of poisons.

HISTORICAL PROGRESSION

Utilizing biology and chemistry, we have progressed significantly since 2000 B.C. when diseases were treated with lizards' blood and toads' eyelids. Trial and error was the driving force until the early 1900s when the effects of crude plants and minerals were analyzed.

The road to pharmacology, as we know it today, was a long and experimental trip traveled by a great many doctors and scientists who did not give up.

During the 100s, Claudius Galen, a noted Greek physician and medical writer, made some findings in anatomy by doing many experiments on both living and nonliving animals. He would strap live pigs or goats to a board to dissect them. He was able to make significant findings using Barbary apes, but said their cries and facial expressions were too human-like to dissect alive. Galen first noted the connection of the larynx to the voice box, the fact that arteries carried blood rather than air, and the discovery that our eyesight is due to the optic nerve. Although he, too, had incorrect theories, his books guided physicians for years. Thanks to people like Galen, today we know a great deal about what causes diseases and illnesses; we also have significant knowledge about cures using drugs.

MEDICINE

Medicine, the science and art of healing, seeks to save lives and relieve suffering. A **drug** is any chemical substance that affects body function. The words *drug* and *medicine* are frequently interchanged. Although tremendous strides have been made in recent centuries, we have a long way to go to fully understand how the human body works and what causes disease. With disease, there is an abnormality of the body regardless of how one feels. When we become ill or have something irregular in our body, we often look to drugs for answers. The more we learn, the more we realize how complicated and complex the human body is. Many of us are aware of the strong connection between the body and the mind. Our thoughts and emotions greatly impact our physical health, but it is rare that our good thoughts alone totally cure us or our bad thoughts alone kill us.

SUPERSTITION VERSUS MODERN MEDICINE

The field of medicine has progressed from superstition and guesswork to a scientific art focusing on mathematics, biology, and chemistry. The first prescriptions were said to be written on stone tablets and long scrolls that date back to 1,000 years before the pyramids were built. Before the nineteenth century, doctors, medicine, and pharmacology were one and the same. Most prescriptions were mere plant remedies until the early 1500s when minerals, lead, and mercury were introduced. Digitalis, a well-known drug used today for heart conditions, was initially used as a sedative and used to treat epilepsy and tuberculosis. Many people died before it was found that digitalis was deadly when administered in high dosages. Because digitalis rids the body of fluid, the intestines were squeezed dry upon overdose. The modern digitalis is called digoxin (Lanoxin). Although digitalis is frequently used today, it is always under watchful doctor's orders. Rarely a day passes when we do not read of new advancements, improved techniques, and new theories of drug administration.

THE PHARMACIST

While it is the physician who diagnoses and prescribes medication, it is the pharmacist who truly understands the drugs (see Figure 1-1). Drug dosages, toxicity, and side effects are the pharmacist's specialty. Because the pharmacist cannot diagnose, pharmacology and the medical field overlap, each relying greatly on the other. In early America, those desiring to be a pharmacist needed the same educational elements we need today: time and money. There were no schools, educational financing, or laboratories. Classes were usually held in rented rooms at night. Even those willing and able to achieve a diploma often did not, largely due to the fact that one did not need any education to obtain a pharmacy license in America until 1932, when it was decided to make the pharmacy course a 4-year course. In 1960, it was increased to a 5-year course.

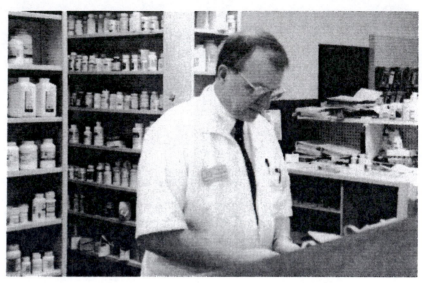

FIGURE 1-1 The pharmacist

MEDICAL MILESTONES

Age 45 was the average life expectancy 100 years ago. Thanks to modern medicine, that has since doubled to 80 to 90 years today. Reasons for that are included in the medical milestones listed in Table 1-1.

NECESSARY CHANGES IN PHARMACOLOGY

In hindsight, we know that a large number of ancient drugs were basically useless. Continued research enables us to build on past limited knowledge to find answers to today's complex medical problems. Because everyone's body is different and reacts differently to the environment, stress, and drugs, there is a constant demand for education,

TABLE 1-1

1899	aspirin introduced
1910	chemotherapy discovered
1922	insulin discovered
1928	penicillin introduced
1938	Dilantin (for epilepsy) introduced
1930s to 1940s	our best germ-fighting drugs came into use
1955	polio vaccine introduced
1960	birth control pills introduced
1970s to present	cancer causes investigated, gene therapy introduced, laser procedures expanded, transplanting of organs, genetic engineering, life-sustaining equipment, cloning, and fetal tissue advancements

growth, and changes in pharmacology. In fact, we probably have as great a challenge in pharmacology today as our forefathers had.

REASONS DRUGS ARE PRESCRIBED

Six Purposes of Drug Therapy

Medications are prescribed for a variety of reasons. Drugs may be ordered to:

1. *Keep healthy people healthy* (see Figure 1-2). Vitamins and insulin are examples of health maintenance medications.
2. *Treat and relieve symptoms.* Over-the-counter medications, such as ibuprofen and aspirin, are used for these purposes (see Figure 1-3).
3. *Prevent certain conditions.* Flu shots, birth control, and vaccines are examples of prophylactic medicine.
4. *Alter normal body processes.* At times we choose to take oral contraceptives or hormones; examples include OrthoNovum 7/7/7 and Estrace.
5. *Reach a diagnosis.* Dyes and barium are aides in helping to diagnose medical problems.
6. *Treat a disease process.* Once a diagnosis is confirmed, the disease process can be treated with antianxiety drugs and antibiotics.

Regardless of why drugs are prescribed, it is essential that regulations and safety guidelines be strictly adhered to.

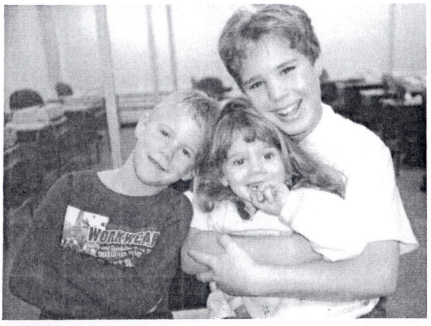

FIGURE 1-2 Health maintenance medications keep healthy people healthy

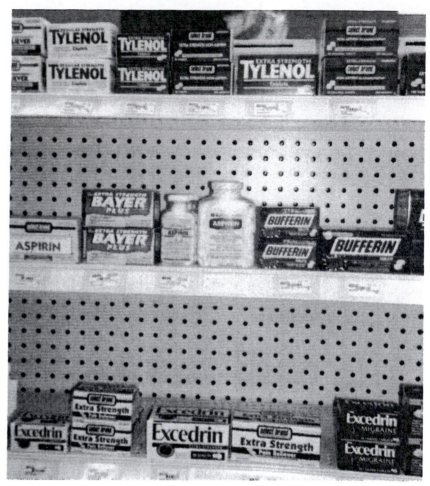

FIGURE 1-3 Over-the-counter medications

MEDICAL/CLERICAL POSITIONS

The Role of the Medical Secretary/Transcriptionist

Competent medical office personnel are one of the physician's greatest assets. Despite the fact a medical secretary/transcriptionist will never prescribe or administer medications, you will be regularly working with drug names, dosages, frequencies, routes, and effects.

IMPORTANCE OF ACCURACY

Accuracy in medical transcription is imperative (see Figure 1-4). You are transcribing a progress note on a patient with a duodenal ulcer when the physician mumbled while dictating the medication. Did the physician dictate "Xanax" or "Zantac"? Does it matter? Should you immediately question the physician or can you determine which medication is correct? The answer is Zantac; it certainly *does* matter! The forthcoming chapters provide the information you need to determine the correct medication. Unless you are absolutely positive that you have correctly

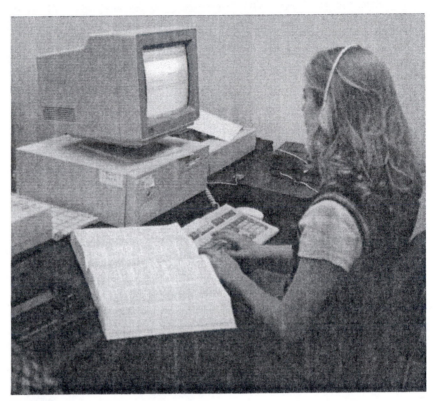

FIGURE 1-4 Medical transcription

identified the medication in question, you need to consult with the dictating physician.

CHAPTER REVIEW

Vocabulary Review

Define the following:

1. pharmacology _____

2. pharmacodynamics _____

3. toxicology _____

4. medicine _____

5. drug _____

Short Answer

6. Explain how modern medicine has changed since the nineteenth century. _____

_____

_____

_____

_____

7. Describe educational requirements for a pharmacist. _____

_____

_____

_____

_____

8. List the six purposes of drug therapy and provide an example. ____

_____

_____

_____

_____

9. Name five medical milestones. _____

_____

_____

_____

_____

10. Explain the importance of accuracy when transcribing medications.

_____

_____

_____

_____

2

Regulatory Agencies, Safety Guidelines, and Controlled Substances

INTRODUCTION

Everyone who directly or indirectly works with medications must understand the requirements that go along with marketing and administering drugs.

As a branch of the U.S. Government, the Food and Drug Administration (FDA) is responsible for maintaining the control and accountability of all drugs prepared and administered. The labeling and the quality of all marketed drugs are overseen by this administration. The FDA promulgates rules and regulations to enforce specific mandates of statutes.

This chapter covers the Drug Enforcement Administration's responsibility and how regulations are met through the Controlled Substances Act (CSA) and why it is important to pharmaceutical companies.

Definitions and characteristics of chemical, generic, and trade names of drugs are covered in detail. Through various learning activities, the reader will practice categorizing controlled substances.

FOOD AND DRUG ADMINISTRATION (FDA)

The drug agency responsible for maintaining and regulating the safety of drugs is the Food and Drug Administration (**FDA**), a division of the Department of Health and Human Services of the U.S. government. The federal Food, Drug, and Cosmetic Act governs the regulations of legalized drugs. Drugs must be validated for safety and proven to be effective *prior* to marketing. Adverse effects of drugs must also be reported to the FDA by the pharmaceutical manufacturer. Even after the FDA has granted approval, this watchdog agency may remove drugs from the market as it deems necessary.

AMERICAN PHARMACEUTICAL ASSOCIATION (APhA)

In 1852, the American Pharmaceutical Association (**APhA**) was founded. The APhA is not a regulatory agency, but a national organization that seeks to maintain the highest standards of practice among its members. This society of pharmacists represents the interests of pharmaceutical professionals and assists members in improving their skills. Because it is strictly voluntary, not all pharmacists choose to belong. The committee is active in pharmacy policy development, public education, publishing, and research.

PUBLIC SAFETY

Stringent regulations protect the public by ensuring the safety and effectiveness of drugs and therapeutic devices. Often drugs are approved, marketed, and in use for 8 to 12 years in other countries before the FDA gives authorization for use in the United States. In America, it is not unusual for it to take years for a new drug to gain FDA approval and become available for consumer use. Despite obvious advantages, critics charge that the "wait" period for new drugs is too long.

NEW DRUGS LIST

Once a drug has been released by the FDA, it may be included in the **New Drugs** list. *New Drugs* is an annual publication by the Council on Pharmacy of the American Medical Association (AMA) to provide health professionals with a current listing of new drugs. Drugs are listed in the *New Drugs* publication until they are granted final approval by the FDA and are included in the *U.S. Pharmacopoeia/National Formulary (USP/NF)*. This formulary, the official source of drug standards, is published approximately every 5 years and details each drug approved by the federal government, listing its standards for purity, composition, strength, uses, dosages, and methods of storage. The NF portion of this formulary specifically lists the chemical formulas of the drugs. Strict standards must be met prior to inclusion in this publication. At this time the new drug is considered "official." When a pharmaceutical company is granted FDA approval for a new drug, it is given a patent preventing another company from manufacturing an identical drug.

PRESCRIBING PROFESSIONS

Once on the market, a clinical physician or dentist is able to prescribe the medication; however, not all physicians can prescribe drugs. Pathologists and doctors in research cannot write prescriptions (unless they choose to be specially licensed).

THE PHARMACY

The drug is prepared, compounded, and dispensed for medical use in a **pharmacy** (see Figure 2-1). The actual compound is prepared by a professional called a **pharmacist** (see Figure 2-2). A pharmacist must obtain a minimum of a bachelor's degree from an accredited institution, complete a 1-year internship program (working under direct supervision of a practicing pharmacist), and successfully pass a state board examination to achieve the registered pharmacist (RPh) credentials.

CONTROLLED SUBSTANCES

Controlled substances are medications that have the potential for addiction and abuse if taken without close supervision by a physician.

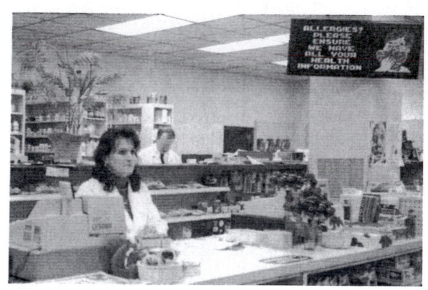

FIGURE 2-1 The pharmacy

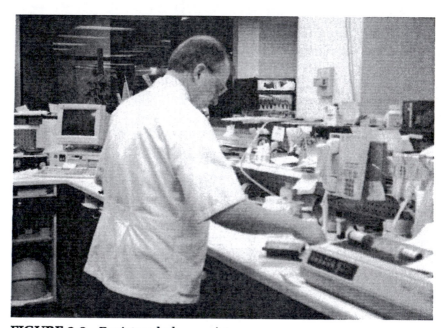

FIGURE 2-2 Registered pharmacist

Stringent federal controls have been designed to minimize the availability of controlled substances and to diminish the opportunity for addiction and abuse.

DRUG ENFORCEMENT ADMINISTRATION (DEA) AND CONTROLLED SUBSTANCES ACT (CSA)

An important date for drug legislation was May 1, 1971, when the **Controlled Substances Act (CSA)** of 1970 became effective.

This act requires all medical practitioners who will have an occasion to dispense, prescribe, or administer a controlled substance to have a narcotic license granted by the **Drug Enforcement Administration (DEA).** Physicians must complete registration to renew this license by June 30 of each year. The DEA number issued appears on all narcotic prescriptions the physician writes. The DEA was established to regulate the manufacturing and dispensing of these dangerous and potentially abused drugs. The Controlled Substances Act sets tight controls on narcotics (drugs that depress the central nervous system, thus relieving pain and producing sleep), stimulants (drugs which increase activity of the brain and other organs), and psychedelics (drugs that produce visual hallucinations such as LSD). A **depressant** is defined as any agent or drug that reduces the function or activity of a body system such as a sedative or anesthetic.

DRUG CATEGORIES

One specific portion of the Controlled Substances Act established a way to classify all drugs into one or more of five categories decided by a predetermined set of criteria based on their potential for causing physical and/or psychological dependence. Schedule II to V drugs have accepted medical use, while Schedule I drugs have no accepted medical use in the United States. All drugs in categories I, II, and III lead to some degree of drug dependence. A few examples in each category have been provided in Figure 2-3.

SCHEDULE OF NARCOTICS

Controlled substances fall into one or more of the five categories as determined by the Controlled Substances Act. Alcohol and tobacco are not included as controlled substances. Refer to Figure 2-4 for examples listed by category.

CONTROLLED SUBSTANCE STORAGE

In health care settings (excluding pharmacies) all controlled substances must be stored separately in a metal compartment, double-locked, properly labeled, and packaged to display the drug's assigned schedule number.

ASSIGNED SCHEDULE NUMBER

The Schedule roman numeral is enclosed in an uppercase "C," indicating the assigned schedule number as shown in Figure 2-5.

DOCUMENTATION

Detailed documentation must be maintained in the health care setting each time a controlled substance is administered. For example, in a

Schedule I

- High potential for abuse
- No accepted medical use in the United States. (There are some circumstances, however, when qualified medical researchers order a synthetic derivative of marijuana as an antiemetic for patients receiving cancer treatment. There are also some eye disorders that are treated with the derivative. When Schedule I drugs are ordered, a DEA form must be completed by the physician ordering the drug.)

  Examples: Lysergic acid diethylamide (LSD); phencyclidine (PCP, angel dust); mescaline and peyote (Mexc., buttons, cactus); methaqualone (quaaludes, ludes); crack (rock); heroin (smack); street-grade cocaine (coke, flake, snow); and marijuana

Schedule II

- High potential for abuse
- Limited medical use in the United States with some restrictions
- A new prescription must be written and a new DEA form completed by the physician each time a Schedule II drug is ordered.
- Severe physical and/or psychological dependence may occur.

  Examples: Narcotics and amphetamines (speed, uppers, crystal, bennies, wake-ups, pep pills); cocaine; codeine; opium; morphine; Demerol; Percodan; pentobarbital; quaaludes; secobarbital

Schedule III

- Some potential for abuse
- Accepted medical use in the United States
- No DEA form is required.
- Moderate/low physical and high psychologic dependence may occur.

  Examples: Narcotics and some barbiturates; various drug combinations containing codeine such as Tylenol with codeine and Fiorinal with codeine; and paregoric glutethimide

Schedule IV

- Low potential for abuse
- Accepted medical use in the United States
- Moderate/low physical and/or psychologic dependence

  Examples: Sedatives and tranquilizers; phenobarbital; Valium; Darvon; Librium; diazepam; and Xanax

Schedule V

- Low potential for abuse
- Accepted medical use
- May be sold over-the-counter in some states
- Limited physical and/or psychological dependence

  Examples: Lomotil; Donnagel; and drugs containing low-strength codeine like cough syrup with codeine.

FIGURE 2-3

Narcotics

Drug	Schedule	Street Names
opium	II, III, V	Dovers powder
morphine	II, III	Miss Emma, Morpho
codeine	II, III, V	School boy
heroin	I	H, Harry, junk, brown sugar, smack
hydromorphone	I	lords
meperidine	II	doctors
methadone	II	dollies

Depressants

Drug	Schedule	Street Names
barbiturates	II, III, IV	downers, barbs
benzodiazepines	IV	
chloral hydrate	IV	Mickey Finn
methaqualone	I	ludes
glutethimide	III	
other depressants	III, IV	

Hallucinogens

Drug	Schedule	Street Names
mescaline; peyote	I	Mexc
phencyclidine	II	PCP, angel dust
LSD	II	
amphetamine variants	I	Ectasy, love drug
other hallucinogens	I	

Stimulants

Drug	Schedule	Street Names
cocaine	I, II	coke, flake, snow
crack	I	rock
methamphetamine	I	ice, crank, crystal
amphetamines	II	uppers, pep pills
other stimulants	III, IV	

Cannabis

Drug	Schedule	Street Names
marijuana	I	grass, joint, pot, Mary Jane, reefers
hashish	I	hash

FIGURE 2-4

FIGURE 2-5 Symbol for a Schedule III Drug

supervised setting such as a long-term care facility, a record of all scheduled drugs must be maintained with thorough documentation of each dosage administered. Regulations dictate how frequently narcotics must be counted, but they should be inventoried at least once a day. Signatures verifying accuracy are required by two authorized individuals.

OVER-THE-COUNTER (OTC) DRUGS

Not all medications require a physician's order. The FDA also regulates **over-the-counter (OTC)** drugs, which are considered safe providing the consumer follows the label directions and heeds the warnings (see Figures 2-6 and 2-7). Chapter 11 covers OTC drugs in more detail.

DRUG NAMES

Chemical Name

There are three methods in which drug names can be assigned. Every drug has a unique **chemical name,** determined by its precise chemical description and molecular structure. The chemical name is made up of letters and numbers, such as octahydro-3; chemical names are not commonly used by a physician's office.

Generic Name

The pharmaceutical company and the U.S. Adopted Names (USAN) Council then determine its **generic name.** Generic names are given to drugs before the drug becomes official. They are written in all lowercase letters and a generic drug may be manufactured by any pharmaceutical company. Examples include tetracycline, procaine, and gentamicin. The patent initially issued includes time spent on research testing and mar-

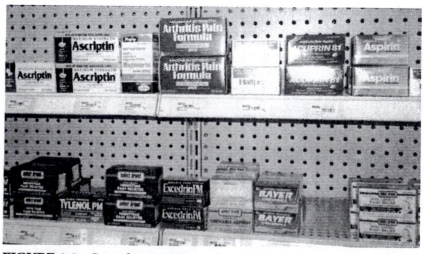

FIGURE 2-6 Over-the-counter medications

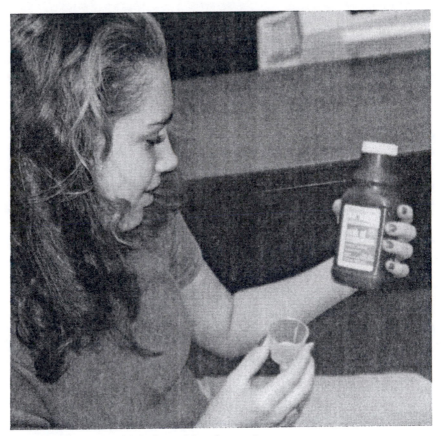

FIGURE 2-7 Read labels and heed warnings

ket trials. When a drug's patent has expired, a generic equivalent can be manufactured by any pharmaceutical company.

Brand Name

Once the FDA gives final marketing approval, most manufacturers select a **proprietary (trade) name** or **brand name** for the drug, requiring a registered trademark (® or ™). The ® indicates the trademark has been registered with the U.S. Patent and Trademark Office, whereas the ™ indicates a trademark but it is not federally registered. The first letter of all trade names is capitalized—Lomotil, Mellaril, and Valium. Often pharmacies carry several brands of the same generic drug. Trade name drugs are more costly as the manufacturer must recoup the initial investment made in developing and testing the drug.

COST EFFECTIVENESS

A major concern in health care is cost effectiveness. Patients are demanding containment of medical care costs. Most health insurance plans pay for generic drugs, whereas brand drug coverage is scrutinized much more closely. The current trend of modern medicine is to treat the patient with the most cost-effective product. This may be obtained by the use of generic substitution or in some formularies, the use of therapeutic substitutions. The only difference between a generic drug and a brand name drug are fillers or dyes. They contain the same active ingredients.

GENERIC DRUG EFFECTIVENESS

Generic drugs will work as effectively as brand name drugs. In some states a pharmacist may substitute a generic drug for a trade name drug unless the physician instructs otherwise. If the physician orders a *specific* trade name drug and writes DAW (dispense as written), only that drug can be dispersed. Most basic categories of drugs are manufactured in a generic form. Refer to Figure 2-8 for examples of generic and trade name drugs.

TRADE NAME SPELLING

There are a number of reasons for the particular spelling of trade names (refer to Figure 2-9).

Generic Name	Trade Name(s)
ampicillin	Amcill, Polycillin, Totacillin
penicillin VK	Pen Vee K
hydralazine hydrochloride	Apresoline
phenytoin	Dilantin
propranolol hydrochloride	Inderal
diazepam	Valium

FIGURE 2-8

- To make spelling and pronunciation easier:

Generic Name	Trade Name
haloperi**dol**	Haldol
pseudoephedrine	Sudafed
erythro**mycin**	E-mycin

- To indicate the drug's source:
    from a **pregnant mare's urine** = Premarin
- To indicate the drug's duration:
    a **slow** release of potassium (**K**) = Slow-K
- To indicate the drug's action:
    to **ascend** the patient out of depression = Asendin
    to **elev**ate the patient out of depression = Elavil
- To indicate ingredients:
    Tylenol #2 contains 15 mg of codeine
    Tylenol #3 contains 30 mg of codeine

FIGURE 2-9

The more familiar you become with drugs, the more apparent the name derivation will become.

CHAPTER REVIEW

Definition

Define the following abbreviations:

1. FDA _____

2. APhA _____

3. DEA _____

4. CSA _____

5. OTC _____

Write the definition of the following terms:

6. *New Drugs* List _____
_____
_____
_____
_____

7. controlled substances _____
_____
_____
_____
_____

8. narcotics _____
_____
_____
_____
_____

9. stimulants _____
_____
_____
_____
_____

10. psychedelics _____
_____
_____
_____
_____

11. Name the two professions that can prescribe medications. _____

_____

_____

_____

_____

12. Explain why not all physicians can prescribe medications. _____

_____

_____

_____

_____

13. Describe safe storage of controlled substances. _____

_____

_____

_____

_____

14. Explain the differences between chemical, generic, and trade name drugs. _____

_____

_____

_____

_____

15. Of the three drugs listed in number 14, which one is the most cost effective? Explain. _____

_____

_____

_____

_____

3

Drug Sources and Forms

COMPETENCIES

At the end of this chapter, the student should be able to:

1. Name the four drug sources and give an example of each.
2. State who is responsible for indicating the form in which a drug may be administered.
3. Differentiate among the three drug forms.
4. Name the four types of solid preparations.
5. Explain why some tablets are scored.
6. Name the three types of semisolid preparations.
7. Give examples of liquid preparations.
8. Name four forms of solutions.
9. Define abbreviations related to the forms of medication.
10. Explain the difference between ointments and creams.
11. Differentiate between a solute and a solvent.
12. Explain how transdermal patches work.

CHAPTER CONTENT

Drug Sources
Drug Forms
   Solid Preparations
   Semisolid Preparations
   Liquid Preparations
   Implantable Devices

INTRODUCTION

Drugs date back to primitive times, when treatment was dominated more by spiritual beliefs than sophisticated modern-day technology. Despite the twentieth century explosive advances in medicine, drugs are obtained from the same four sources today as they were historically. There have, however, been many recent changes in the form by which a drug can be administered. In order to accurately transcribe physicians' orders and follow through with ordering medications, the medical assistant, medical transcriptionist, and medical secretary must understand the various forms by which a drug can be administered.

DRUG SOURCES

A drug can be obtained from four different sources.

- *Plants.* Crude drugs may be obtained from various parts of plants—leaves, roots, fruit, bark, or herbs. Plants for medicinal purposes date back to primitive cultures when it was thought the use of herbs evoked magical powers. Examples of drugs derived from plants include morphine, derived from opium; and poppy and digoxin, from *Digitalis lanata.*

- *Animals.* Numerous essential extracts are obtained from animal tissue. Drugs are then produced from the extracts, such as the hormone insulin (from the pancreas of cows or hogs used to treat diabetes) and lanolin (from sheep's wool used as an ointment base). Cortisone (an anti-inflammatory agent) is extracted from the adrenal glands of animals and is also a hormone (from the thyroid gland of animals) used to treat rheumatoid arthritis. Insulin is now also produced synthetically by pharmaceutical companies.

- *Minerals.* From magnesium, the antacid/laxative Milk of Magnesia (MOM) is derived. Iron and iodine are other nonorganic substances of the earth's crust. Sulfur is a mineral which has been used for many years as an antibacterial agent. Sulfa drugs are now synthetically manufactured and are used to treat urinary tract infections and intestinal infections.

- *Synthetics.* Tremendous advancements have been made in recent years in pharmaceutical laboratories creating compounds, either artificially or as a result of a natural process. Synthetics were produced not only to save money, but for those allergic to products made from animal tissue, plants, and minerals. Examples include the analgesic meperidine (Demerol), the antidiarrheal diphenoxylate (Lomotil), as well as several other antibiotics and narcotics. By synthetically producing medications, they can be produced in significant quantities and are much more economical. Recently, through a technique called *gene splicing*, scientists have created new strains of bacteria. Humulin, an insulin used to treat diabetes, is an example of genetic engineering which will likely revolutionize the pharmaceutical world in years to come.

In order to obtain FDA approval, the pharmaceutical company must indicate the form(s) in which the drug may be administered. Drugs must be taken in the correct form in order to be effective. There are basically three forms of drug administration: solids, semisolids, and liquids.

Solid Preparations

Solid preparations include tablets, capsules, caplets, and lozenges. (Occasionally powders are included as a fifth type of solid preparation as seen in chapter 5.)

Tablets (tabs). A tablet is a single-dose, disk-like unit containing dried medicinal powdered drugs prepared in a mold. Examples include aspirin and Naprosyn.

- Enteric Coating. Some tablets are covered with a protective coating (**enteric coating**) to prevent their absorption in the stomach. Dissolving of the special coating occurs in the small intestine, preventing stomach irritation. Examples of enteric tablets include Advil, Motrin, and Thorazine. See Figure 3-1 for an example of an enteric tablet.
- Layered/Long-Acting. Layered tablets, containing two or more layers of the same or different ingredients, provide different absorption rates over a several hour span; hence, **long-acting (LA)** forms. The LA abbreviation is usually part of the trade name, indicating a sustained-release drug. An example is Entex LA.
- Scored. Some tablets are scored, making it convenient for the patient to break them into halves or quarters to vary the dosage.

Examples of scored tablets include Reglan, CalanSR, and Duricef (see Figure 3-2).

Capsules (caps). Capsules are a powdered drug within special containers made of gelatin. They may contain two hard shells which fit together and hold the ingredients in place. The container prevents the patient from tasting the drug. Examples include Benadryl and Axocet (see Figure 3-3).

- Spansule (Spans). This is a registered trademark of the SmithKline pharmaceutical company, that designates a slow-release (SR) capsule. Medication disburses gradually. An example is Compazine Spansules.

FIGURE 3-1 Enteric tablet.

FIGURE 3-2 Scored tablet.

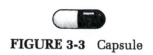

FIGURE 3-3 Capsule

Caplets. Caplets are similar in size and shape to a capsule; however, they are coated and have the consistency of a tablet for oral administration. Examples include Tylenol Cold Severe Congestion and Nuprin (see Figure 3-4).

Lozenges (troche). Lozenges are solid, usually flat, round preparations, not swallowed but dissolved in the mouth, releasing the drug topically into the tissue of the mouth and throat. Examples include cough drops and Cepacol (see Figure 3-5).

Semisolid Preparations

Semisolid preparations include suppositories, ointments, and creams.

Suppositories (supp). A suppository is a semisolid base of soap, glycerinated gelatin, or cocoa butter containing a drug for introduction into the rectum, vagina, or urethra, where it dissolves when subject to body heat. **Suppositories** are labeled "for external use only" and are usually lubricated with a water-soluble jelly for easier insertion (see Figure 3-6). Examples include Thorazine and Monistat.

Ointment (ung). An ointment is a semisolid, medicated emulsion of water globules in a fat base for external topical application. The **ointment** is applied with a rubbing stroke for antiseptic, cosmetic, or healing properties. Examples include Ben-Gay and Kenalog (see Figure 3-7).

FIGURE 3-4 Caplet

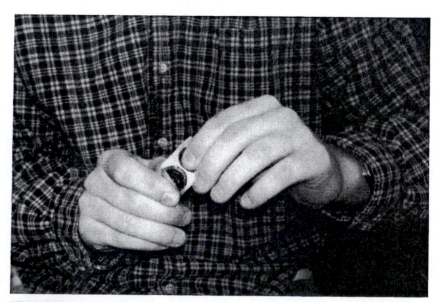

FIGURE 3-5 Lozenges

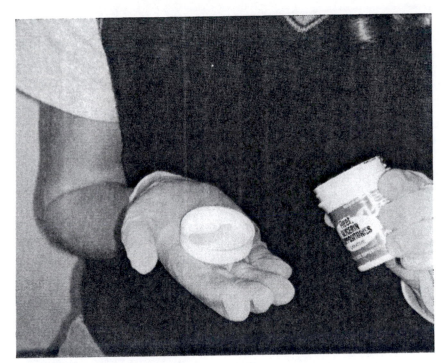

FIGURE 3-6 Suppositories

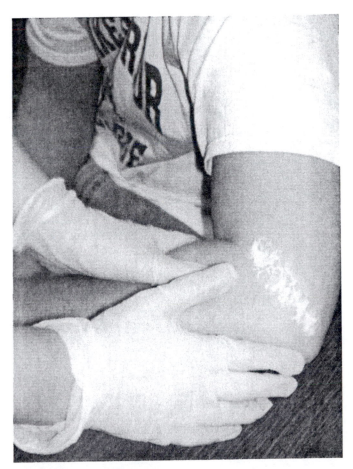

FIGURE 3-7 Ointment

Cream. A cream is a semisolid emulsion (a mixture of two liquids not mutually soluble) of fat globules in a water base. A **cream** is prepared for local external application (see Figure 3-8). Examples include hydrocortisone cream and Topicort cream.

Liquid Preparations

Liquid preparations contain drugs dissolved or suspended and when taken internally (with the exception of emulsions), are rapidly absorbed through the stomach or intestinal wall. Not all liquid preps are to be ingested. The following are types of liquid preparations.

Solutions (sol). A solution consists of one or more substances completely dissolved. Each solution has two parts. The **solute** is the dissolved substance, and the **solvent** is the liquid in which the solute is dissolved. Examples include Condylox and Ocean.

Various forms of solutions include:

- Elixirs—Elixirs contain alcohol, sugar, water, and occasionally a flavoring to disguise the bitter taste of the drug. Common users include children and the older population. Examples of elixirs include phenobarb elixir, Tylenol elixir, and the elixir of Donnatal. Elixirs are also available in other drug forms.
- Syrup (syr)—Syrups contain sugar, water, and flavorings, but no alcohol. They may or may not contain medicinal additives, and are thicker than elixirs. Examples include Ipecac syrup and cough syrup (see Figure 3-9).
- Tincture (tinct)—An alcoholic extraction of vegetation or animal substance. An example is tincture of iodine.
- Suspension (susp)—The state of a solid when its particles are mixed with, but not dissolved in, a fluid. These liquids must be well shaken before administered. Examples include Maalox and Milk of Magnesia (see Figure 3-10).

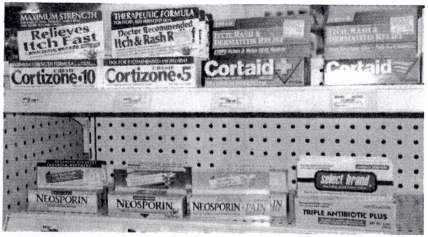

FIGURE 3-8 Cream

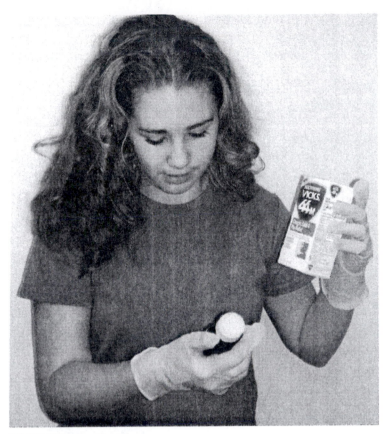

FIGURE 3-9 Cough syrup

- Lotion—An active drug in a water base for local external application; it should be patted on. Examples include Caladryl lotion and Keri lotion.
- Liniment—A drug used externally that produces a feeling of heat when massaged on a given area. An example is methyl salicylate.

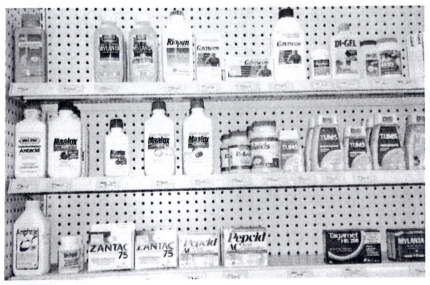

FIGURE 3-10 Maalox suspension

- Aerosol—Aerosols are packaged as a pressurized unit that may include ointments, creams, lotions, medications, powders, or liquids (see Figure 3-11). Examples include Azmacort™ and Mycelex.
- Spray—Sprays are administered by an atomizer and are frequently used for nose and throat treatment (see Figure 3-12). An example is Neo-synephrine.

Emulsions. **Emulsions** are fine droplets of either oil in water or water in oil. They must be vigorously shaken to ensure mixing prior to use. An example is castor oil.

Drops (gtt). Drops are a liquid medication usually instilled in ears and eyes. Examples include Murine and Neodecadron.

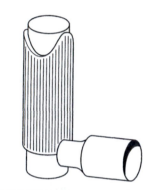

FIGURE 3-11 Aerosol spray

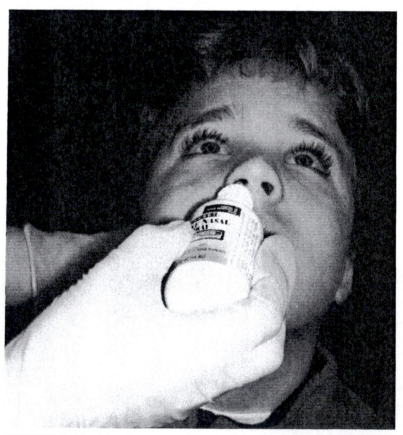

FIGURE 3-12 Nasal spray

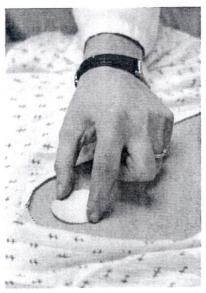

FIGURE 3-13 Transdermal patch application

Transdermal Patch

A transdermal patch, used to administer medication to a targeted area, is a fairly recent method of drug delivery (see Figure 3-13). These multi-layered disks contain a drug reservoir. The adhesive layer holds the "patch" on the skin. Between the drug reservoir and the skin is a thin, porous membrane. The tiny holes control and regulate the amount of drug released into the bloodstream in a consistent manner over a given period of time. The impermeable backing prevents the drug from leaking out to the surrounding areas. Transdermal patches are often used to reduce motion sickness in automobile and air travel (Transdermscop), relieve nicotine withdrawal symptoms (Nicoderm and Habitrol), and relieve chest pain (nitroglycerin).

Implantable Devices

There are several devices available for implantation just beneath the skin. The blood vessels provide a direct lead to the desired area to be medicated. These devices have been proven successful for birth control and chemotherapy treatment. One example is Norplant.

CHAPTER REVIEW

Short Answer

1. Name the four drug sources. _____

_____

_____

_____

_____

2. Provide an example of a drug derived from each drug source.

_____

_____

_____

_____

_____

3. List four examples of solid preparations. _____

_____

_____

_____

_____

4. Explain why a tablet may be scored. _____

_____

_____

_____

_____

5. List three examples of semisolid preparations. _____

_____

_____

_____

_____

Abbreviations

Provide the appropriate abbreviations for the following:

6. tablet _____

7. capsule _____

8. suppository _____

9. ointment _____

10. solution _____

11. drops _____

12. syrup _____

13. suspension _____

14. long-acting _____

15. Spansules _____

Essay

Define or explain the following words/phrases:

16. The difference between a solute and a solvent. _____

_____

_____

_____

_____

17. The difference between an ointment and a cream. _____

_____

_____

_____

_____

18. Explain why emulsions must be shaken. _____

_____

_____

_____

_____

19. Describe how a transdermal patch works. _____

_____

_____

_____

_____

20. List two reasons why a device might be implanted. _____

_____

_____

_____

_____

Drug Dosages and Effects

At the end of this chapter, the student should be able to:

1. Match age groups with the appropriate categories.
2. Describe the difference between local and systemic effects.
3. Describe the steps necessary for an ingested medication to be effective.
4. Provide examples of local and systemic applications.
5. Differentiate between a therapeutic dose, maintenance dose, maximal dose, and lethal dose.
6. Define pharmacology terminology.
7. Define drug effect terminology.
8. Define therapeutic index, adverse effect, and toxic effect.
9. Describe the manufacturer's responsibility regarding side effects.
10. Name four of the eight undesirable effects of drugs.
11. Differentiate between drug addiction and drug abuse.
12. Explain drug interaction with certain foods, beverages, or other medications.

CHAPTER CONTENT

Drug Dosage
Factors Influencing Effectiveness
   Gender
   Age and Weight
   Physical Conditions
   Drug Interaction
   Prophylaxis
   Synergists and Antagonists
Body's Response to Drug Administration
Steps to Drug Effectiveness
   Absorption
   Distribution

INTRODUCTION

In an ideal world, there would be a one-pill panacea (cure-all) for every sign, symptom, disorder, and diagnosis. This pill would cure the condition without causing any undesired effects or adverse reactions.

Unfortunately, we do not live in an ideal world. By understanding the actions of a drug, sometimes the effects—both positive and negative—can be predicted. This chapter helps the medical assistant, medical transcriptionist, and medical secretary better understand drug dosages, the desired effects of drugs, and some of the problems that can arise from drug administration.

DRUG DOSAGE

The word **dosage** refers to the amount of medication to be administered. No medication is 100 percent effective for each person who uses it. To avoid unwanted interactions, the physician must know all medications the patient is taking including nonprescription products. It is important to keep in mind that not all conditions or diagnoses require a prescribed medication.

FACTORS INFLUENCING EFFECTIVENESS

In a health care setting, only authorized personnel can legally administer medication. The overall effectiveness of medication is dependent on several factors. Factors that must be considered prior to prescribing a medication include the patient's gender, age, weight, physical condition, other prescribed medications, and the most appropriate method of administration. In addition to these factors, the individual prescribing the drug must be cognitive of any patient allergies or drug sensitivities.

Gender

Some medications react differently in men than women and vice versa. Along with the patient's gender, hormones, genetic makeup, and differences in the rate of body metabolism can alter the overall effectiveness of medications.

Age and Weight

Not all medications are appropriate for all age groups. Although age is an important consideration when prescribing medications, the patient's weight is equally important. As an example, a medication would affect a 5'2" 13-year-old who weighed 90 pounds differently than a 6'2" 18-year-old who weighed 210 pounds (see Figure 4-1).

Although you will find differences in opinions and some age overlapping, patients are usually divided into the following age groups:

Newborn: 0–4 weeks
Infant: 5–72 weeks
Child: 1–16 years
Adolescent: 12–18 years
Adult: 18–60 years
Geriatric: 60 years and older

Physical Condition

When ordering medications, the physician must take into account if the patient is pregnant or breast feeding, has drug allergies, or is grossly

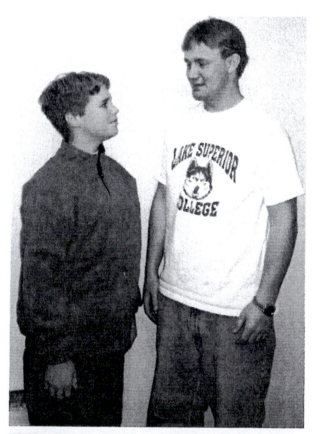

FIGURE 4-1 Age and weight influencing factors

obese. These are the major factors that must be contemplated prior to a medication being prescribed.

Drug Interaction

It is not uncommon for a patient to be taking two prescription drugs at the same time. New federal requirements mandate the pharmacist provide patients with counseling regarding drug effects, dosages, frequency, forms, and food and drug compatibility. Mixing some medications with certain foods, beverages, or other medications can increase or decrease the effectiveness of the drug and can produce a dangerous or even fatal crisis.

Prophylaxis

Some medications have a **prophylactic** action, tending to ward off or prevent disease, such as vaccines.

Synergists & Antagonists

One drug can favorably enhance the effect of another drug. Drugs which react favorably together are known as **synergists.** Others have undesirable effects—they can produce an unfavorable response by heightening side effects. Undesirable effects are called **antagonists.** Also, a drug's effect can be enhanced or diminished by ingestion of some foods.

Figure 4-2 lists commonly used drugs that could cause trouble if mixed with the wrong substance. *It is not recommended to take alcohol with any prescribed medication.*

To reiterate, as some medications act as antagonists, the physician should be aware of all medication the patient is taking, both prescription and over-the-counter.

BODY'S RESPONSE TO DRUG ADMINISTRATION

While one drug may only have one route, another may have several. The physician determines the route best suited for the patient.

STEPS TO DRUG EFFECTIVENESS

To be effective, once the chemical substance is in the body, it must be absorbed, distributed, metabolized, and excreted.

Absorption

Absorption enables the drug to be distributed into the bloodstream. The rate of absorption is dependent on factors like the route of administration, the drug administered, and the condition of the individual, including age and weight.

If you take . . .	Don't mix medications with . . .
acetaminophen	alcohol
antibiotics	fatty foods
anticoagulants	cholesterol reducers, thyroid medications, alcohol, aspirin
anticonvulsants	folic acid, Antabuse
antidiabetics	aspirin, alcohol
antifungals	alcohol
antigout	aspirin
antihistamines	alcohol (causes drowsiness and slows reactions), major tranquilizers
blood pressure pills	chickenpox, flu, asthma, gout, ulcers, bleeding disorders; do not take with alcohol or fruit juice
bronchodilators	alcohol, tranquilizers
ibuprofen	aspirin allergy, asthma, heart failure, ulcers, kidney problems; do not take on an empty stomach
naproxen sodium	alcohol, aspirin, allergy, pregnancy, asthma, heart failure, kidney problems, ulcers
painkillers	sedatives, tranquilizers, alcohol
penicillin	a full stomach as it reduces absorption into your system
sleeping pills	alcohol
tetracycline	milk, cheese, or ice cream; if pregnant, do not take with iron preparations
tranquilizers, major	alcohol, antihistamines, barbiturates, or any other tranquilizer
tranquilizers, minor	sedatives, antidepressants, alcohol
vasodilators	foods high in salt

FIGURE 4-2

Distribution

Once in the bloodstream, the chemical substance is distributed into body tissues and/or body fluids and transported to the intended site. The physical properties and the composition of the chemical substance determine how this distribution is made. The medication undergoes a chemical alteration leading to its breakdown to allow for elimination.

Metabolism

The physical and chemical alterations that occur in the body are collectively known as **metabolism.** Metabolism refers to all the chemical operations occurring in the body. As an end result of the metabolic operations, unneeded or potentially harmful waste products must be eliminated.

Excretion

The last step in the process is **excretion,** or when the drug is eliminated from the body. The waste products of the chemicals can be excreted from the body system in a number of ways. Excretion takes place in the kidneys through urine, in the skin through perspiration, in the respiratory tract through mucus, in the digestive tract in bile and feces, and through the reproductive tract in breast milk.

LOCAL AND SYSTEMIC EFFECTS

The effect a drug has upon a body is divided into two categories. Drugs act either locally or systemically. A **local effect** is limited to the immediate area where the medicine is applied. This can be accomplished by:

1. applying a drug topically, such as rubbing methyl salicylate on painful joints;
2. injecting the drug under the skin; or
3. injecting the drug into a nerve to provide anesthesia.

Examples of local application include ointments containing anti-inflammatory agents and antibiotic agents, most rectal and vaginal suppositories, enemas, nasal sprays, and ear preparations (see Figure 4-3). These are covered in more detail in chapter 5.

A **systemic effect** is felt throughout the patient's body. This is accomplished by the drug being absorbed or injected into the bloodstream and then distributed throughout the system. To produce a systemic effect, a drug can be taken orally, sublingually, parenterally (describing all methods of administering medications by means of a needle or a cannula—a flexible outer tube that surrounds a sharp, pointed trocar, introduced through the skin (see Figure 4-4)—rectally, through inhalation (see Figure 4-5), or less frequently, topically. Methods of administering local and general anesthesia to produce systemic effects are covered in more detail in chapter 5.

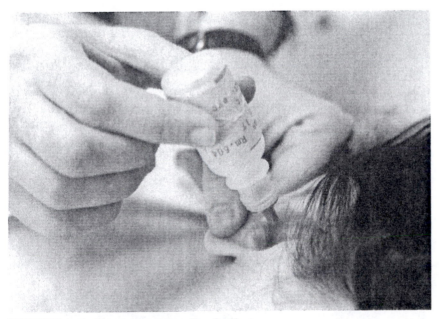

FIGURE 4-3 Ear preparation local effect

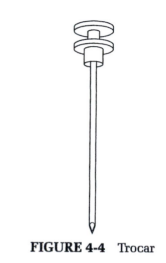

FIGURE 4-4   Trocar

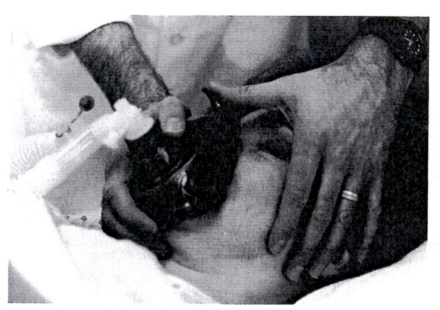

FIGURE 4-5   Inhalation therapy

STANDARD DRUG DOSAGE TERMINOLOGY

Standard terminology used to describe dosages include the following:

- The **initial dose** is the first dose administered.
- The **average dose** is the amount of medication taken to produce effective results with a minimal toxic effect.
- The **therapeutic** (minimal) **dose** is the smallest amount of drug that will produce a desired effect. The **therapeutic effect** is the desired effect that will treat or cure the medical condition.
- A **maintenance dose** keeps concentrations of the drug at a therapeutic level.
- A **maximal dose** is the largest amount of drug that will produce a desired effect without symptoms of toxicity (poisoning). The

therapeutic index is the range between the minimal and maximum dosages. Some medications are premeasured and individually packaged in a per-dose basis termed *unit dose.*

UNDESIRABLE DRUG EFFECTS

Ideally, every drug administered would cure the disease for which it was prescribed, therefore causing no ill effects. Unfortunately, this is not always the case. Occasionally, a drug will cause an undesirable action or an effect other than the one for which the drug was prescribed. Some of these highly undesirable actions include side effects, adverse effects, toxic effects, lethal doses, allergic reactions, anaphylactic shock (which is life threatening), habituation, addiction, and drug abuse.

Side Effects

Side effects, the mildest of these undesirable effects, are usually mild and short-lived. The FDA requires the manufacturer to develop and provide a complete listing of common side effects prior to marketing a drug. This list must also be made available to the consumer when obtaining the drug. Common side effects include nausea, vomiting, dizziness, wheezing, shortness of breath, itching, hives, eye redness, and diarrhea. These are usually short-lived and subside in a reasonable period of time. There is no need to contact a physician unless they do not subside or they become severe. More severe effects include blood in the urine, severe abdominal pain, or uncontrollable emotional outbreaks.

Adverse Effects

When a side effect becomes severe, it is referred to as an **adverse effect.** These unfavorable and potentially harmful effects are one of the leading causes of emergency room visits in the older population. Contact the physician if common side effects persist for an extended period of time. *The physician must be contacted immediately* if a patient experiences any severe side effects.

Toxic Effects

A **toxic effect** results when the serum level of a drug rises beyond the therapeutic level to a level of toxicity. A **toxic dose** is the amount of a drug that would cause signs of drug toxicity. Physicians order blood tests to monitor drug levels for patients on medications known to frequently cause toxic effects. A common example would be when a patient is on the blood thinner Coumadin.

Lethal Doses

A **lethal dose** is a drug amount that could or does cause death.

Allergic Reactions

Patients occasionally exhibit a hypersensitivity (idiosyncrasy) commonly known as an **allergic reaction** to medications. A mild reaction is characterized by itching, swelling, wheezing, and sneezing.

Anaphylactic Shock

A severe reaction can include bronchospasm and shock. A life-threatening allergic reaction is termed *anaphylactic shock.*

Habituation, Addiction, and Drug Abuse

Three other undesirable drug effects are habituation, addiction, and abuse. **Habit-forming** drugs cause a psychological craving, rather than a physiologic dependence when a drug is withheld. It is difficult to differentiate between **habituation** (becoming accustomed to taking a drug or a psychological dependence) and addiction (a physical and/or psychological dependence).

An **addiction** is when the body becomes physically and/or psychologically dependent (also termed physiologically dependent) on the abused drug. The drug becomes essential to the maintenance of normal cellular activity. When there is a drug addiction, there is often a tendency to increase the drug dosage to obtain a desired effect because the body develops a **tolerance** to the substance and more of the drug is needed to achieve the same effect that was accomplished with a smaller amount previously. The four major groups of substances that frequently cause addiction include:

1. narcotics,
2. sedatives and tranquilizers,
3. amphetamines, and
4. alcohol.

Refer to chapter 11 for more information and examples of drugs falling into these categories.

Drug abuse is the harmful, nonmedical use of a mind-altering drug. Regardless of the drug involved, the tell-tale signs of continual misuse and drug abuse are the same:

- Mood swings
- Health, behavior, attitude, or personality changes
- Poor muscle coordination
- Slurred speech
- Unusual sleepiness or restlessness
- Unexplained absences from home, work, or school

To prevent the preceding list of problems, it is imperative the physician be aware of *all* drugs, prescription and nonprescription, that the patient is taking.

CHAPTER REVIEW

Definition

Define the following:

1. dosage _____

2. absorption_____

3. distribution _____

4. metabolism_____

5. excretion_____

Short Answer

6. List six factors necessary for effective medication ingestion._____

_____

_____

_____

_____

7. Describe the difference between a synergist and an antagonist. ____

_____

_____

_____

_____

8. Define a local effect._____

_____

_____

_____

_____

9. List the ways a drug can be administered to produce a systemic effect. _____

_____

_____

_____

_____

10. Differentiate among side effects, adverse effects, and toxic effects.

_____

_____

_____

_____

11. Match the following definition with the correct letter.

a. lethal dose
b. average dose
c. therapeutic dose
d. maintenance dose
e. therapeutic effect

f. initial dose
g. maximal dose
h. therapeutic index
i. unit dose
j. toxic effect

_____ 1. Individually packaged in per-dose basis.

_____ 2. The first dose administered.

_____ 3. Keeps concentrations at a therapeutic level.

_____ 4. The smallest amount of drug that will produce a desired effect.

_____ 5. The largest amount of drug that will produce a desired effect without toxicity.

5

Routes, Methods, and Documentation of Medication Administration

COMPETENCIES

At the end of this chapter, the student should be able to:

1. List the five main routes of drug administration.
2. Name the six "rights" of drug administration.
3. Name the four forms of oral solid medication.
4. Name the advantages of oral administration.
5. Name the disadvantages of oral administration.
6. Name the ways liquid medication can be measured.
7. Describe the two special types of topical administration.
8. Explain the three types of IV injections.
9. Differentiate between general and local anesthetics.
10. Name two common general anesthetics.
11. Give two methods of administering local anesthetics.
12. Describe inhalation therapy.
13. Explain uses of inhalation therapy.
14. Name three most commonly used syringes.

CHAPTER CONTENT

Routes of Administration
> *Oral Administration*
> *Sublingual Administration*
> *Buccal Administration*
> *Topical Administration*
> *Parenteral Administration*
> *Other Parenteral Injection Sites*

Patient Responsibility
Universal Precautions
Six Rights of Drug Administration
Documentation Guidelines
Medication Errors

Anesthesiology
General Anesthesia
Local Anesthesia

INTRODUCTION

It cannot be too strongly emphasized that medical secretaries, medical receptionists, medical coders, and medical transcriptionists cannot legally administer drugs. Medical assistants, with proper training, may administer medications. However, most medical office personnel will be working with drug names, dosages, frequencies, and routes of administration on a day-to-day basis.

It is imperative you know the proper route by which a medication would be administered. When transcribing physicians' dictation, it is often difficult to differentiate between two drugs that sound alike. In some instances, the transcriptionist can accurately determine the correct medication by verifying the route of the drug. This chapter explains routes of drug administration and gives examples of each method. Injections and the equipment used are also covered. You must be familiar with the types of anesthetics administered and the terminology that goes along with them.

Pharmaceutical preparations are designed for specific routes of administration.

Medications are administered through particular routes to achieve specific results. Just as some drugs can be dispensed in more than one form, some drugs can be administered by more than one route. The effect of a drug is dependent on the route of administration.

ROUTES OF ADMINISTRATION

There are various ways to categorize the most common routes of administering drugs. You will find reference books differ; some refer to only two routes: the GI tract and the parenteral. Others consider each method of administration as a separate method of delivery. These have been outlined in two ways but elaboration was provided specifically on Example 2, which is often considered the five main routes of drug administration.

Routes of Administration: Example 1

    I. GI Tract
      A. Oral
      B. Nasogastric
      C. Rectal
    II. Parenteral
      A. Sublingual
      B. Buccal
      C. Injections
        1. intradermal

2. intramuscular
3. intravenous
4. sub-Q
D. Topical
1. transdermal (transcutaneous)
E. Inhalation

Routes of Administration: Example 2

I. Oral
II. Sublingual
III. Buccal
IV. Topical
    A. Instillation
    B. Inhalation
V. Parenteral
    A. Sub-Q
    B. IM
    C. IV
    D. Intra-arterial, intraosseous, intrathecal

The five main routes of administration from Example 2 are defined in detail as follows.

Oral Administration

Taking a medication by mouth is the most common, convenient, economical, and acceptable method, and is the best for self-administration. It is a relatively easy and safe method of administration in that the skin is not broken, as it is with injections. Ordering a medication by mouth is abbreviated p.o. (Latin for "per os" meaning "by mouth"). Examples of medications taken orally include aspirin and Tylenol.

Solid and liquid forms. Oral medications can be administered in a solid or liquid form (see Figures 5-1 and 5-2). Solid forms include tablets, capsules, caplets, lozenges, and sometimes powders. When a medication is administered in a liquid form, it is normally measured by fluid ounce (fl oz), cubic centimeter (cc), milliliter (ml), teaspoon, or tablespoon. In addition to the teaspoon and tablespoon, three measuring devices—a medicine cup, a standard water cup, or a calibrated medicine dropper, can be used. Regardless of the measuring device, measurement accuracy is essential. In order to visualize cubic centimeters in comparison to fluid ounces and milliliters, Figures 5-3, 5-4, and 5-5 may be helpful.

Advantages of oral administration. There are advantages to taking oral medication in a liquid form. One advantage is that a liquid may be easier to swallow than pills. Another advantage is that, when appropriate, drugs with an unpleasant taste may be disguised in a fluid such as fruit juice or a syrup.

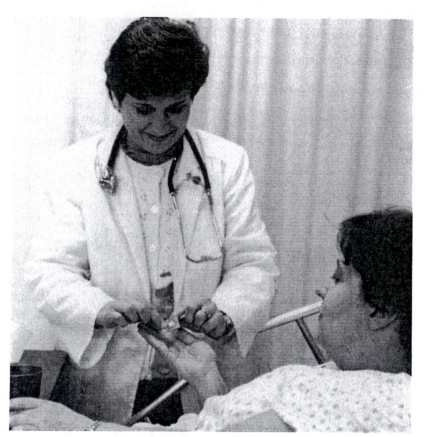

FIGURE 5-1 Oral medication in solid form

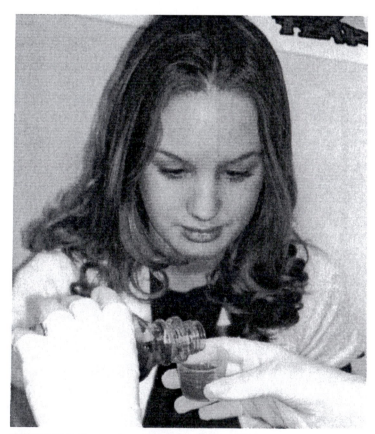

FIGURE 5-2 Oral medication in liquid form

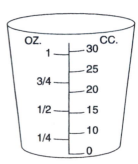

FIGURE 5-3   Fluid ounces versus cubic centimeters

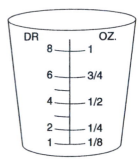

FIGURE 5-4   Drams versus ounces

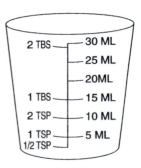

FIGURE 5-5   Teaspoon/tablespoon versus milliliters

Disadvantages of oral administration.   Disadvantages of oral administration include the fact that they are slower to act than other routes because they must be absorbed in the GI system before being effective. They may also cause an irritation of gastric mucosa. Some drugs, such as certain antibiotics, are inactivated or altered by digestive enzymes; thus, they should not be given orally. Other drugs are unsuitable for oral administration because they are insoluable or poorly absorbed. The oral methods are not always suitable for infants, small children, those comatose or dysphagic, or patients with frequent vomiting.

Sublingual Administration

Sublingual medications are placed under the patient's tongue, where they are retained until dissolved and absorbed. The drug can be in the form of tablets or liquid. Because the drug is rapidly and completely absorbed through mucous membranes and the large blood vessels under the tongue, it has a much faster therapeutic effect than the oral method. This route allows lower dosages to be given than with oral medications, therefore minimizing potential side effects. When a rapid onset of action is needed, such as relief of chest pain, the antianginal medication nitroglycerin is administered sublingually.

Buccal Administration

In **buccal** (pertaining to the cheek) **administration,** a medication is held between the gum and the cheek. Similar to sublingual administration, the drug (usually a tablet) dissolves against the mucous membrane (transmucosal). Mycelex troche is an example of buccal administration. A disadvantage of absorption through mucous membranes is that eating or drinking may interfere with the medication's effect.

Topical Administration

Another common method of administration is **topical,** where the drug is applied directly to the skin on a specific area of the body or into an easily accessible body cavity. The active drug in a topical preparation must be in a vehicle that allows the drug to be released and diffused through the skin such as vaginal creams, hemorrhoidal preparations, suppositories, or oral analgesic creams designed to treat a local area. Topical preps are specifically formulated and packaged in unit-dose patches which provide a precise amount of drug released over a specified time. Patients often find this application very convenient. Transdermal patches vary in size and shape as illustrated in Figure 5-6. Topical preps include ointments, creams, powders, lotions, liniments, and tinctures. Two special types of topical administration include drug instillation and inhalation.

Instillation. Instillation involves the application of a drug into body cavities such as the conjunctival sacs of the eyes, ears, nose, throat, vagina, and rectum. Mucous membranes in these areas are generally more permeable than the skin, as discussed in the transdermal drug form section in chapter 3. Absorption rate is dependent on the vascularity and the thickness of the specific membrane. In general, instillation can provide both systemic and local effects.

- *Eyes.* Ophthalmic medications offer a local effect when administered using the proper technique (see Figure 5-7). If not administered properly, the medication can flow into the lacrimal duct and upon being absorbed can cause a systemic effect.
- *Ears.* Ear preps are instilled into the ear canal using the instillation method (see Figure 5-8). Otic medications are used to treat inflammation and infections, as well as to dislodge foreign bodies and to soften cerumen.
- *Nose.* Nasal medications are administered by instillation in the form of drops, or by a nasal spray (see *Inhalation*).
- *Throat.* Sprays are drugs prepared to such a consistency that they may be administered by an atomizer. Some drugs administered using this method function as astringents producing a shrinking or contracting effect.
- *Rectal and vaginal.* Rectal administration includes suppositories, ointments, and enemas. Rectal suppositories are often inserted for

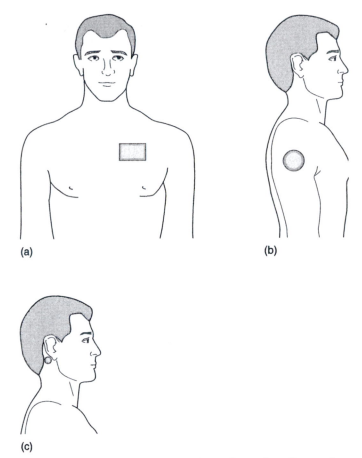

(a)

(b)

(c)

FIGURE 5-6   (a, b) illustrate dermal patches for angina pectoris; (c) is a patch to prevent motion sickness

laxative purposes. They offer fast-acting relief of constipation by promoting normal peristalsis throughout the large intestine. Suppositories can provide systemic relief and are also used as analgesics, antipyretics, antiemetics, and anti-inflammatory agents. Enemas safely and effectively produce colonic peristalsis when fluid is introduced just past the internal anal sphincter. Enemas are used to cleanse the lower bowel to prepare patients for x-rays and various diagnostic and surgical procedures. Vaginal administration is in the form of suppositories, creams, or tablets.

Inhalation.   Inhalation, the second type of topical administration, is the introduction of dry or moist air, or medicated vapor or gas (O_2, CO_2, or helium), through the mouth or nose into the lungs for therapeutic purposes. This requires special apparatus such as respirators to deliver positive-pressure breathing, inhalers, nebulizers, humidifiers, and some nasal sprays (see Figure 5-9 (a–d) for samples of these types of equipment). Hand-held inhalers are aerosol units containing medication which produce a fine mist that is inhaled to facilitate breathing for those with chronic obstructive pulmonary disease (COPD). Inhalers can be oral or nasal, dependent on the physician's order. The oral inhaler is often used by patients with asthma and the nasal inhalers are frequently ordered for local treatment of nasal congestion. An example of a systemic effect is a

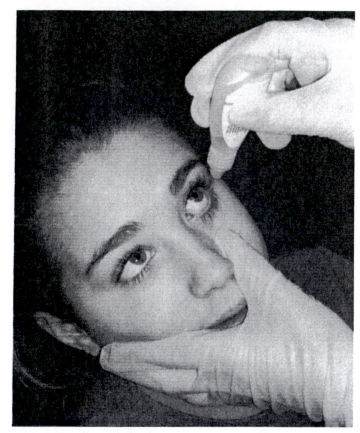

FIGURE 5-7 Ophthalmic medication offers local effect

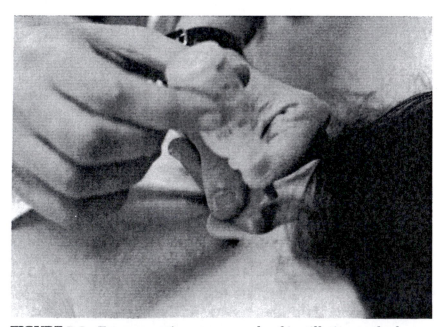

FIGURE 5-8 Ear preparation one example of instillation method

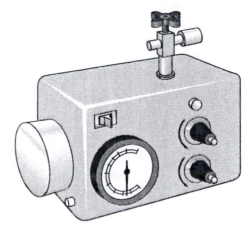

FIGURE 5-9 (a) Respirator to deliver IPPB

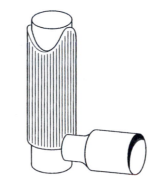

FIGURE 5-9 (b) Metered-dose inhaler

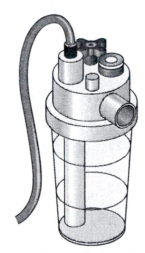

FIGURE 5-9 (c) Nebulizer

vasopressin derivative administered for nocturnal bed-wetting. Two examples of inhalation therapy are provided in Figures 5-10 and 5-11.

Extreme caution must be exercised when patients are receiving oxygen therapy, both by the patient and those interacting directly with the patient. Because oxygen is highly combustible, there is to be absolutely *no* smoking or smoking material in the area where oxygen is

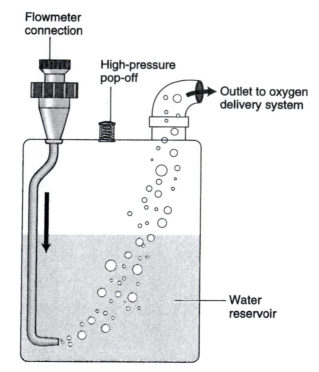

FIGURE 5-9 (*continued*) (d) Bubble humidifier

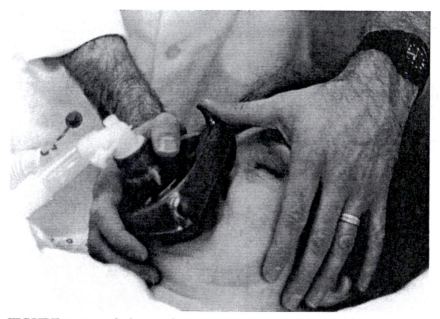

FIGURE 5-10 Inhalation therapy (mask)

being administered. When oxygen is stored, the tanks must be securely fastened in a nonpatient area.

Inhalation can provide both local and systemic effects. Intranasal preps, used as decongestants or used as bronchodilators for asthma, provide local relief. Face masks or endotracheal tubes are used routinely to induce general anesthesia to produce a systemic effect. Disadvantages of this route include the need for careful patient teaching and special equipment for proper administration.

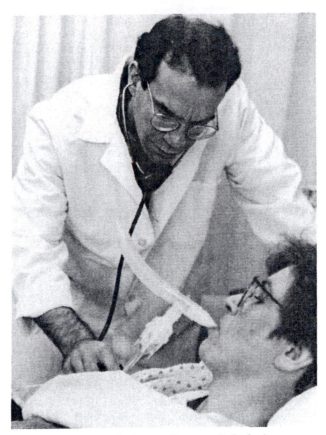

FIGURE 5-11 Inhalation therapy (inhaler)

Parenteral Administration

The word, "parenteral," derived from the Greek language, translates to "apart from the intestines." Some reference books define parenteral routes as "any route other than the GI tract." More commonly, it is defined as "a collective term including all ways in which drugs are administered with a needle." The primary advantage of this route is the rapid absorption of a precisely measured amount of drug. The most common types—subcutaneous (sub-Q), intramuscular (IM), and intravenous (IV)—are described in detail later in this chapter.

Parenteral administration is the most rapid, direct, and effective route. There are three significant advantages of parenteral administration.

1. Patient's mental and/or physical condition could make it difficult or impossible for the patient to take a medication orally, buccally, or by any other route.
2. Parenterally administered medications do not enter the digestive system and are, therefore, not altered by digestive acids or enzymes.
3. Medications can be targeted to provide direct effects in one specific area.

Although there are advantages of the parenteral route, there are also disadvantages. Despite the use of sterile equipment and drug solutions, whenever the skin is broken there is a risk of infection. There is always the risk of penetrating a nerve, a blood vessel, or striking a bone. If not administered accurately, a sub-Q or IM medication could be injected intravenously, or an IM injection could be given subcutaneously. Another disadvantage is that it allows little or no margin for error, as once it is administered, it is virtually irretrievable, and allergic reactions can range from mild to fatal. Although there are advantages of the parenteral route, it can also be hazardous.

Injection equipment. Equipment used for injections includes syringes, vials, and ampules.

Syringes have a variety of uses and come in all sizes. They can be glass or plastic, prepackaged, sterile, assembled or unassembled. Uses include administering drugs, adding sterile solutions to IV flasks, and irrigating wounds, eyes, or ears. Most syringes and needles are disposable to prevent cross-infection and cross-contamination.

All syringes have three parts: the *tip* (can connect to a **needle**), the *barrel* (holds medication or other substance and has preprinted calibrations, and the *plunger* (the tight-fitting movable part which fits inside the barrel) (see Figure 5-12). The size and calibrations vary according to how the syringe will be used (see Figure 5-13).

The most commonly used syringes for parenteral use are the standard syringe, tuberculin syringe, and the insulin syringe.

A *standard* (or regular) *syringe* is an instrument for injecting liquids into or withdrawing them from any vessel or cavity. The standard syringe that holds up to 3.0 ml is usually calibrated with two scales, ml (cc) and minims. The larger standard syringe is calibrated in milliliters only. A standard hypodermic syringe is usually of small caliber to administer drugs in a solution or other liquid. The injection is made through a hollow needle of small bore into the subcutaneous tissues. The size and calibration is dependent on the syringe's typical use. The 3 cc size (0.1 calibration) is for IM and sub-Q injections (see Figure 5-14). The 5 cc size (0.2 calibration) is for a venipuncture and IV injections (along with 10, 20, and 50 cc calibrations). The larger sizes—10 cc, 20 cc, and 50 cc— are for medical and surgical treatments, aspirations, irrigations, and stomach feedings.

The *tuberculin* syringe is especially calibrated in hundredths of a milliliter on one side (see Figure 5-15) and minims on the other side (0.1 and 0.01 calibrations) for small, precise measurements in intradermal and allergy injections, and for allergy testing. The TB syringe has both the metric and apothecaries' scales on the barrel.

The **insulin syringe** is similar to the hypodermic, except the calibrated scale is in "units" especially designed for insulin, commonly 50 U or 100 U (see Figure 5-16). The insulin syringe is the only one to have the needle permanently attached and no dead space (does not allow for fluid to remain in the needle or syringe after the plunger is depressed

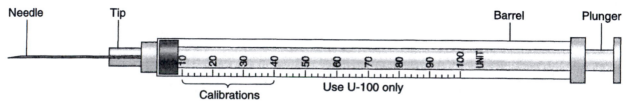

FIGURE 5-12

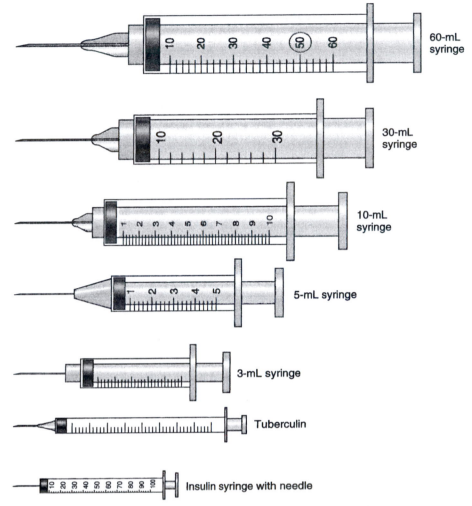

FIGURE 5-13   Various sizes of disposable syringes and calibrations

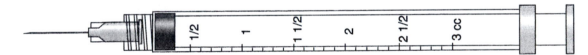

FIGURE 5-14   Standard syringe cc/mL

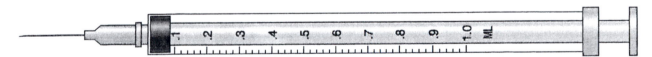

FIGURE 5-15   Tuberculin syringe

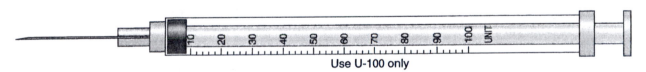

Use U-100 only

FIGURE 5-16   Insulin syringe

fully). These are specially designed for self-administration of the correct amount of insulin.

You will find syringes used today are classified as either disposable or nondisposable. The disposable syringes are sterile, prepackaged, durable plastic. They are often preferred for parental medication administration; they are safer, save time, and are less expensive than nondisposables. Some disposable syringes can be purchased *prefilled*. Pre-filled are the most convenient, but are also more costly than disposables that are filled by the person administering the drug. Disposable syringes are packaged in sealed, rigid plastic containers or in peel-apart paper wrappers. Those administering the injection must use extreme care when disposing of any syringe-needle unit. Nondisposable syringes are made of strengthened glass and are frequently used for procedures such as thoracenteses, thoracotomies, and tracheotomies.

Just as there are disposable and nondisposable syringes, there are disposable and nondisposable needles as well. Those administering injections must be aware of the differences and know how to select the appropriate syringe and needle and the necessary precautions to take with the disposal of each. Disposable syringes with used disposable needles are to be discarded in biohazardous puncture-proof containers (see Figure 5-17).

Medications to be injected are supplied either in vials or ampules. **Vials** are small, sterile, pre-filled glass bottles with a sealed rubber-stopper on the top, designed for multiple withdrawals. **Ampules** are small, sterile, prefilled glass containers usually designed for one-time usage (see Figures 5–18 and 5–19). Once opened, the ampule cannot be resealed; the unused portion is to be immediately discarded. Ampules are used for IV emergency drugs such as epinephrine (Adrenalin) and 50% dextrose (D50).

Types of injections
- **Intradermal:** With intradermal injections, the needle is inserted almost parallel with the skin surface (see Figure 5-20(a). This method is used for administering skin tests (Mantoux and tine tests) and for allergy testing.

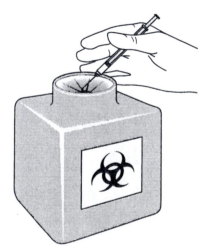

FIGURE 5-17 Biohazardous puncture-proof container

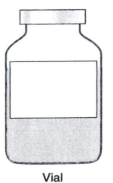

Vial

FIGURE 5-18

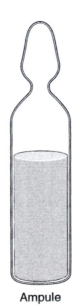

Ampule

FIGURE 5-19

- **Subcutaneous (sub-Q) injections:** The liquid is injected under the skin into the adipose layer between the dermis and the layer of muscle. The proper positioning of the needle for sub-Q injections is at a 45 degree angle. Compare the angles between the intradermal and sub-Q injection positions (Figure 5-20a, b).

  Adipose tissue has a diminished blood supply so drugs are absorbed more slowly by the sub-Q route than the IV or IM. Patients who need daily injections, such as insulin-dependent diabetics or those needing regular allergy injections, must rotate the injection sites. Almost any area of the body surface can be used as a site for sub-Q injections, although the most common sites are the lateral aspects of the upper arms, anterior thighs, and the abdomen. Volumes up to l ml may be given sub-Q. The disadvantages of sub-Q injections are minimal, although this route can cause tissue irritation and may be uncomfortable and painful.

- **Intramuscular (IM):** With intramuscular injections, the needle is positioned at a 90 degree angle (see Figure 5-20c). These injections produce a much faster effect than the sub-Q injections. For IM injections in adults, a 1- to 3-inch needle is used to inject up to 5 ml of liquid into the area of the greatest mass (belly) of a

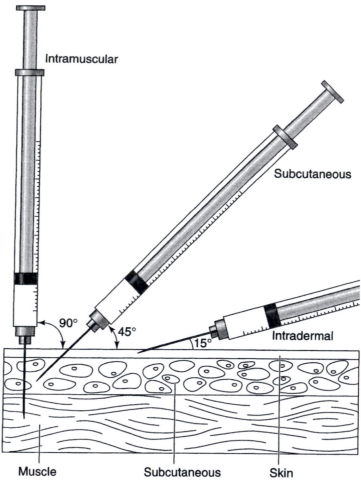

FIGURE 5-20 Needle angles of injections. (a) intradermal;
(b) subcutaneous; (c) intramuscular.

muscle. For children, the injection site and the size of the needle used is determined by the size of the child.

Several sites may be used including the deltoid (upper arm; see Figure 5-21(a) and (b)), vastus lateralis (lateral aspect of the mid-thigh; see Figure 22), rectus femoris (anterior aspect of mid-thigh; see Figure 5-23), the gluteus medius (upper lateral hip area; see Figure 5-24), and the gluteus maximus (upper outer quadrant of each buttock; see Figure 5-25).

When repeated administration of IM injections are ordered, the sites are rotated to minimize pain and reduce numerous injections of the same site. Drugs that are not water soluble will seep out of IM tissue; therefore, the manufacturers recommend they not be given IM. This route can be painful and may cause muscle damage which could increase bleeding risks during anticoagulant therapy.

- **Intravenous (IV):** Intravenous injections provide the most rapid onset of a drug. Medications are administered directly into the bloodstream, or more specifically, into a vein. This is by far the most common way of administering emergency drugs because the medicinal effects are manifested within minutes. The intended effect occurs rapidly because intravenous injections do not

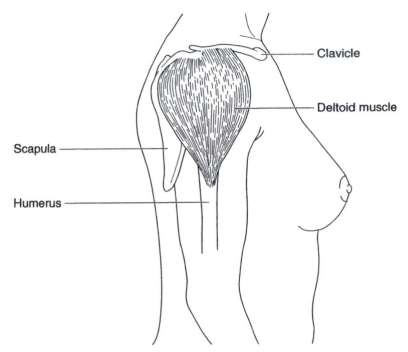

Clavicle

Deltoid muscle

Scapula

Humerus

FIGURE 5-21 (a)   IM injection into deltoid muscle

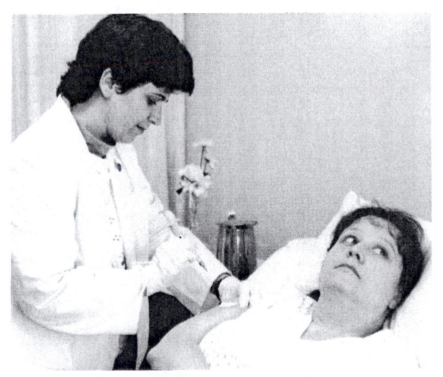

FIGURE 5-21 (b)   IM injection into deltoid muscle

require absorption from tissue or muscle. There is a risk of infection or incompatibility with other drugs, however, and it is not suitable for self-administration. Specialized equipment is needed with IV therapy, which automatically infuses a predetermined amount of fluid into the line. This is measured by so many ml/hr or so many drops/min.

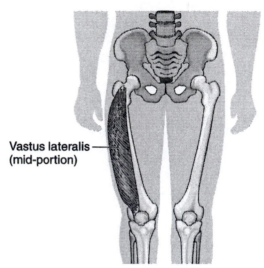

FIGURE 5-22 IM injection into lateral aspect of the vastus lateralis

Vastus lateralis (mid-portion)

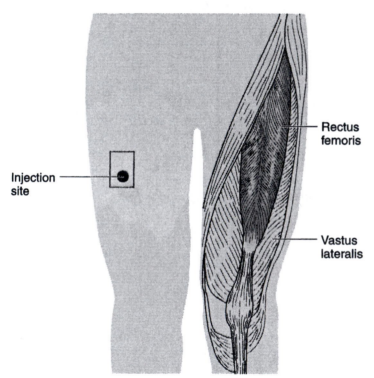

Rectus femoris

Injection site

Vastus lateralis

FIGURE 5-23 Rectus femoris site

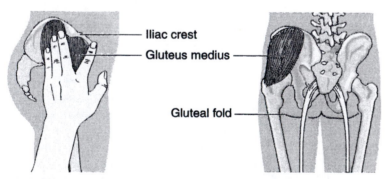

Iliac crest

Gluteus medius

Gluteal fold

FIGURE 5-24 IM injection into gluteus medius

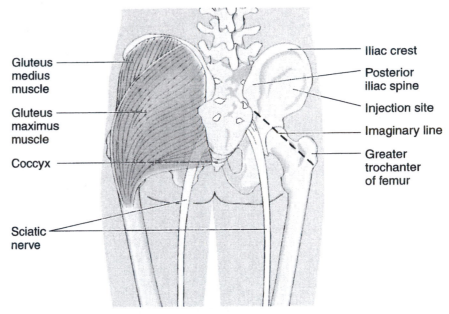

Gluteus medius muscle

Gluteus maximus muscle

Coccyx

Sciatic nerve

Iliac crest

Posterior iliac spine

Injection site

Imaginary line

Greater trochanter of femur

FIGURE 5-25 IM injection into gluteus maximus

Types of IV injections.   There are three types of IV injections:

1. A single dose of a drug (**bolus**) can be injected into an existing IV line through a rubber stopper (port). Because the drug is virtually pushed into the IV line, this method is known as an **IV push.**
2. A drug mixed with a fluid in a bottle or bag that is administered continuously over several hours is an **IV drip** (see Figure 5-26). This provides gradual administration of the drug.
3. The **piggyback** is when a drug is mixed in a very small bag or bottle, and it is connected to a port and administered into the existing IV line to empty within an hour (see Figure 5-27). Drugs given by this method include Valium, antibiotics, or chemotherapy drugs.

IV fluids.   Commonly used IV fluids contain dextrose, electrolytes, or a combination of both. Dextrose acts very similar to glucose upon entering the bloodstream. Those you will hear most often are dextrose 5% in water (D5W) and dextrose 10% in water (D10W). Dextrose 50% in water (D50W) is only used in life-threatening situations such as severe hypoglycemia in diabetics or premature infants. One important electrolyte (a solution capable of conducting electricity) often administered is sodium. This physiologic salt solution is also known as normal saline. Phrases you will often hear are: Normal saline, half normal saline, and dextrose 5% in normal saline.

Other parenteral injection sites.   Less common types of parenteral injections include:

- *Intra-arterial:* A chemotherapeutic agent is injected directly into an artery which leads to the tumor, affected organ, or tissue. This provides rapid results similar to IV administration. Toxic effects can also develop very quickly. Because there are potential dangers

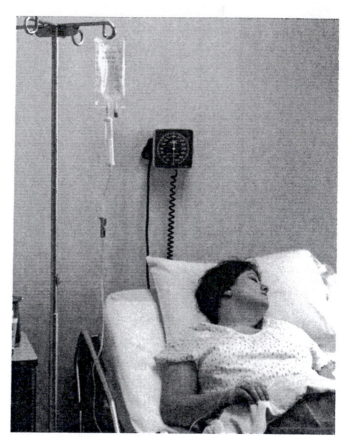

FIGURE 5-26 IV drip

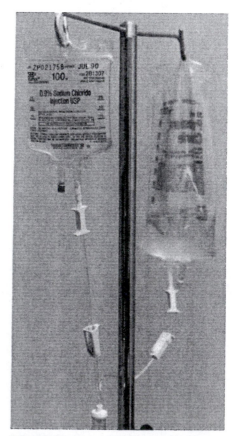

FIGURE 5-27 Piggyback method

with injecting into an artery, extreme caution must be taken when using this route.

- *Intra-articular:* The process of injecting corticosteroids directly into a joint to reduce inflammation or pain.
- *Intrathecal and epidural:* Greek for "within a sheath," an intrathecal liquid is injected into the subarachnoid space around the spinal cord. With an epidural, a drug is injected between the vertebrae into the extradural space. These routes are used when high concentrations of a drug are desired, such as antibiotics for acute nervous system injections or for a spinal anesthetic.

PATIENT RESPONSIBILITY

Pharmacists provide written information on all prescriptions filled; however, the patient must assume responsibility for taking medication appropriately (see the sample Patient Instruction Sheets in Figures 5-28, 5-29, and 5-30). Have you ever taken a capsule for the common cold and washed it down with an alcoholic beverage? Have you forgotten to take a dosage of medication and then doubled the next dose to make up for it? More than 50 percent of those taking medication are guilty of these very dangerous activities. The following is a list of rules for safe administration of medication.

1. Follow directions as written on the label.
2. Do not use medication ordered for someone else. The dosage depends on a patient's age, sex, and physical condition; the dosage may be wrong for you.
3. Do not crush or chew medicine unless the label states to do so. Crushing certain tablets destroys protective coatings that mask bitter-tasting substances. It could also cause the tablet to dissolve before reaching the desired body location, lessening or destroying the effectiveness.
4. "Take on an empty stomach" means 1 hour before or 2 hours after eating. It takes 2 hours for digested food to leave the stomach.
5. If you miss taking a medication at a designated time, do not double the next dose unless the physician or pharmacist authorizes it. Most medications are given in small doses several times a day rather than one large dose once a day in order to maintain the proper blood level for the medicine. In some cases, a double dose could cause a toxic effect.
6. Antibiotics are usually taken for 10 days. Finish the entire prescription even if symptoms subside.
7. Do not use leftover medications.
8. Do not stop using or cut down on a prescribed drug without consulting with your physician.
9. Store medications only in original containers with labels securely attached. Never mix pills in one bottle even if you think you can distinguish between them.
10. A medication should never be taken or administered if there is *any* question regarding the medication order.

```
┌─────────────────────────────────────────────────────┐
│                  ROBERTS CLINIC                      │
│                 3965 YETKA LANE                      │
│               ANYTOWN, MN  55811                     │
│                  218-555-0923                        │
│                                                      │
│                                                      │
│  DATE: 4/23/00                        PAGE:  1       │
│  CUSTOMER: DAHL, KATHY                RX#: 729571     │
│  DOCTOR: JACOB DAVIDSON               REFILLS LEFT: 2│
│                                                      │
│  GENERIC NAME:  TRIAMCINOLONE (trye-am-SIN-oh-lone)  │
│                                                      │
│  COMMON USES:  This medicine is used to reduce       │
│  itching, redness, and swelling which is associated  │
│  with many skin diseases.                            │
│                                                      │
│  HOW TO USE THIS MEDICINE:  Follow the directions    │
│  for using this medicine provided by your doctor.    │
│  TO USE THIS MEDICINE:  Apply a small amount of      │
│  medicine to the affected area. Gently rub the       │
│  medicine in until it is evenly distributed. Wash    │
│  your hands after applying this medicine, unless     │
│  your hands are part of treated area. DO NOT         │
│  BANDAGE OR WRAP the affected area unless it is       │
│  directed otherwise by your doctor. IF YOU MISS A    │
│  DOSE OF THIS MEDICINE, apply it as soon as          │
│  possible. If it is almost time for your next dose,  │
│  skip the missed dose and go back to your regular    │
│  dosing schedule.                                    │
│                                                      │
│  CAUTIONS:  IF YOUR SYMPTOMS DO NOT IMPROVE          │
│  WITHIN A FEW DAYS, or if they become worse, check   │
│  with your doctor. DO NOT USE THIS MEDICINE longer   │
│  than the time prescribed by your doctor. DO NOT     │
│  USE THIS MEDICINE for other skin conditions at a    │
│  later time. DO NOT GET THIS MEDICINE in your eyes.  │
│  IF THIS MEDICINE WAS PRESCRIBED FOR THE             │
│  TREATMENT OF THE DIAPER AREA OF A CHILD, avoid      │
│  using tight-fitting diapers or plastic pants.       │
│                                                      │
│  POSSIBLE SIDE EFFECTS:  CHECK WITH YOUR DOCTOR      │
│  AS SOON AS POSSIBLE if you experience itching,      │
│  burning, redness, or swelling. If you notice other  │
│  effects not listed above, contact your doctor,      │
│  nurse, or pharmacist.                               │
│                                                      │
└─────────────────────────────────────────────────────┘
```

FIGURE 5-28 Patient Information Sheet

11. Never store medication within reach of children. Use childproof caps and keep out of children's reach.
12. All medication must be kept in a safe storage place. Medications stored in a medical facility are to be safely and properly stored away from direct patient access.
13. Depending on the medication, some require refrigeration, others must be stored in darkness (opaque containers), and others must be stored in glass containers.
14. Near your telephone, post the telephone number for Poison Control, your physician, and the nearest hospital.

```
                    ROBERTS CLINIC
                    3965 YETKA LANE
                  ANYTOWN, MN  55811
                    218-555-0923




DATE: 01/03/00                          PAGE:  1
CUSTOMER: DAHL, JAIME                   RX#:  624306
DOCTOR: JACOB DAVIDSON                  REFILLS LEFT:  1

GENERIC NAME:  AMMONIUM LACTATE

COMMON USES:  This medicine is used to treat dry, scaly skin and to
relieve the itching that goes with this condition.

HOW TO USE THIS MEDICINE:  Follow the directions for using this
medicine provided by your doctor.  SHAKE WELL before using a dose.
Apply this medicine to the affected area and rub throughly. IF YOU
MISS A DOSE OF THIS MEDICINE, use it as soon as possible. If it is
almost time for your next dose, skip the missed dose and go back to your
regular dosing schedule.

CAUTIONS:  Do not get this medicine in your eyes or on the inside of
your nose and mouth.

POSSIBLE SIDE EFFECTS:  SIDE EFFECTS, that may go away during
treatment, include mild redness, stinging, or burning where the
medicine is applied. If they continue or are bothersome, check with your
doctor. If you notice other effects not listed above, contact your doctor,
nurse, or pharmacist.
```

FIGURE 5-29 Patient Information Sheet

Often state laws govern who may administer prescription drugs. Individuals preparing or administering medications are ethically and legally responsible for their own actions. These health care professionals are usually certified (as an EMT or CMA), licensed (as an LPN), or registered (as an RN).

UNIVERSAL PRECAUTIONS

The U.S. Department of Health and Human Services offers specific universal precaution guidelines for the prevention of HIV and other blood-borne diseases. These guidelines pertain to health care professionals who may encounter bodily fluids including blood, all body secretions and excretions, nonintact skin, and mucous membranes. For those in the health care field, regardless of the setting, it is essential that universal precautions be practiced every minute of every day.

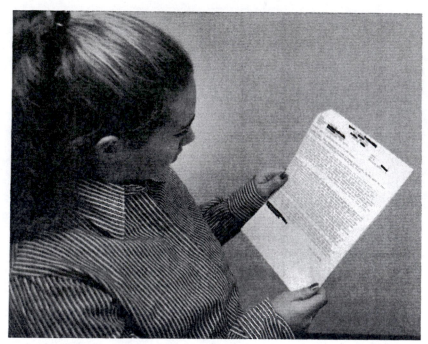

FIGURE 5-30 Patient assumes responsibility for proper medication administration

SIX RIGHTS OF DRUG ADMINISTRATION

Whether you take your own medications or are administered medication, there are six "rights" for proper drug administration to ensure safe delivery.

1. The *right patient*
2. The *right medication*
3. The *right dosage and frequency*
4. The *right route*
5. The *right time of day*
6. The *right documentation*

Each of these are described in more detail below.

1. The *right patient* is checked by asking the patient to state his or her name. For those in an acute care setting, the patient's ID bracelet is checked. The patient may be asked to identify him or herself. It is not advisable to ask the patient if he or she is Mr. or Mrs. Johnson; some patients will answer to any name.
2. To ensure the *right medication* is given, the label on the drug container is to be checked twice before administering the drug and once after the drug has been administered. There should be an allergy check done as well.
3. Again, triple-check the label to verify the *right dosage and frequency*. The dosage ordered and the dose on hand should be the same.

4. To verify the *right route*, double-check the physician's order. If it is parenteral, verify the correct site.
5. Often military time is used for recording the time a medication is administered. When verifying the *right time*, be sure the medication is given at the prescribed interval. Also, check to see if the medication should be given with or without food.
6. For the person preparing and administering the medication, another right to be considered is the *right documentation*. Medication should only be administered by the person who prepared it, and medication should only be prepared by the person who will administer it.

DOCUMENTATION GUIDELINES

There are stringent guidelines regarding the documentation of medication administration. When a medication is administered by an authorized health care worker, the person administering the medication records his or her initials in the appropriate box on the Medication Administration Record. This entry must be made in ink. Observation is necessary to ensure the patient does not experience side effects or adverse reactions. If the patient does experience results other than the desired effect, thorough documentation must be made in the patient's record, with appropriate follow-up according to facility policy.

If a medication is not administered as ordered, again, thorough documentation should be made in the patient's chart with the reason why the medication was not taken.

MEDICATION ERRORS

By using the six rights of drug administration, you can determine when a medication error has occurred. If any or all of the following occur, it is considered a medication error. It is a medication error when the medication administered was:

Given to the *wrong patient*
The *wrong medication*
The *wrong dosage or frequency*
Administered by the *wrong route*
Given at the *wrong time*

The person identifying the medication error must immediately follow the facility's policies and procedures for proper steps to document and rectify the error.

It is possible to administer the correct medication to the correct patient, but make an error in *documentation*. You must follow the facility's policies to make necessary corrections. This type of error is usually not considered a med error, but is a documentation error.

ANESTHESIOLOGY

Anesthesiology is the study of medicine dealing with the absence of feeling, pain, or sensation in all or part of the body. An **anesthetic** is an agent that *causes* that absence of feeling. There are many ways to administer an anesthetic.

General Anesthesia

General anesthesia eliminates pain by inducing unconsciousness, or a total body anesthesia. Frequently, an anesthesia is given to *induce* unconsciousness, and then either a continued IV or inhalation is used to *maintain* the unconscious state. General anesthesia plays an important role in surgery, as it not only eliminates the patient's pain, but also relaxes muscles, making incisions easier for the surgeon. General anesthetic agents used may be inhaled (I) or injected (IM or IV). Some common general anesthetics include:

nitrous oxide (N2O or laughing gas), (I)
chloroform, (I)
ether, (I)
cyclopropane, (I)
thiopental (Pentothal or Pent.), (IV)
halothane (Fluothane), (I)

Local Anesthesia

Local anesthesia is normally injected at or near the region to be anesthetized, or is applied topically. It is given mainly to abolish painful stimulation prior to a minor surgical procedure such as a tooth extraction or an obstetric delivery. A local has the ability to desensitize one specific location. Local anesthetics are rarely given as a systemic analgesia, and are not administered orally as they are inactivated by gastric acids. Examples of local anesthetics include benzocaine, procaine, lidocaine (Baylocaine), and mepivacaine (Carbocaine). Two methods of administering local anesthetics include block and topical.

Block/regional. The goal is to inject the drug agent either near its desired site of action or at the nerve supply to that region. You will often find the word ending "-caine" usually indicates a general or local anesthetic (lidocaine, procaine, and etidocaine). A *spinal or epidural* is a form of a block; however, the drug is injected into the spinal canal or epidural space. It produces a loss of sensation in the lower body, including the legs. Examples include lidocaine (Xylocaine), procaine (Novocain), and tetracaine (Pontocaine). With a *caudal block,* the drug affects the nerves outside the spinal canal. The lower body becomes anesthetized while the patient remains conscious. *Neuromuscular blocks* are given IV which block nerve transmissions inducing skeletal muscle relaxation. Examples include Flaxedil, metocurine (Metubine), and vecuronium (Norcuron). The injection of a local anesthetic that produces a wall of anesthesia around the operative site is known as a *field block*. Acupuncture, the insertion of needles into certain pressure points, can also produce anesthetic results.

Topical or surface anesthesia. Topical or surface anesthesia provides brief periods of insensitivity of the skin. Common types include dibucaine (nupercainal), lidocaine (Xylocaine), tetracaine (Pontocaine), and benzocaine (Solarcaine and Dermoplast).

CHAPTER REVIEW

Place a check mark on the five main routes of drug administration.

_____ 1. parenteral

_____ 2. sublingual

_____ 3. intrathecal

_____ 4. liquid

_____ 5. topical

_____ 6. standard

_____ 7. IM

_____ 8. oral

_____ 9. general

_____ 10. buccal

Short Answer

11. Name the two types of topical administration. _____

_____

_____

_____

_____

12. List three disadvantages of oral administration. _____

_____

_____

_____

_____

13. Explain the differences between a vial and an ampule. _____

_____

_____

_____

_____

14. Describe inhalation therapy. _____

_____

_____

_____

_____

15. Name four body cavities where instillation therapy may be used. _____

_____

_____

_____

_____

16. Explain why extreme caution must be exercised with oxygen (O2) therapy. _____

_____

_____

_____

_____

17. Name two disadvantages of parenteral administration. _____

_____

_____

_____

_____

18. Describe the following parts of a syringe:
tip
calibrations
plunger

_____

_____

_____

_____

19. Explain when tuberculin syringes are used. _____

_____

_____

_____

_____

20. Explain why sites are rotated when IM injections are repeated. ___

___
___
___
___

21. Name 8 of the 14 rules of patient responsibility of safe drug administration. ___

___
___
___
___
___

Define the following abbreviations:

22. cc ___

___
___
___
___

23. ml ___

___
___
___
___

24. COPD ___

___
___
___
___

25. sub-Q ___

___
___
___
___

26. Match the following "right" with the appropriate statement.

_____ a. administer med at 1200 hrs

_____ b. triple-check med label

_____ c. administer IV

_____ d. "no apparent side effects"

_____ e. compare drug container label with order

_____ f. ID bracelet indicates Michael A. Matare #4044

_____ g. med charted by person administering it

_____ h. administer 0.125 mg Lanoxin

1. the right patient

2. the right medication

3. the right dosage and frequency

4. the right route

5. the right time of day

6. the right documentation

Drug Terminology and
Prescription Abbreviations

INTRODUCTION

The medical language used in the health care field, both written and spoken, primarily consists of acronyms, eponyms, and abbreviations. Every individual employed in this field must be familiar with the medical terms used; however, few professions deal more closely with medical terminology than the medical assistant, medical transcriptionist, and medical secretary. These individuals deal with medical terms every time a chart is opened, a progress note or report is transcribed, and a piece of paper is filed into a medical record. To carry out these duties effectively, these individuals must be well-versed in medical terminology and appropriate acronyms, eponyms, and abbreviations.

This chapter provides the material to more clearly understand pharmacology terminology.

In order to better understand this book, there are pharmacology words, phrases, definitions, and abbreviations you must be familiar with. Many words and phrases in this chapter are also included in chapter 11 under the pertinent drug classifications.

DRUG TERMINOLOGY

acetylcholine: A neurotransmitter that plays an important role in transmitting nerve impulses. Its action is blocked by anticholinergic drugs.

addiction: Physical and/or psychological dependence on a substance.

adrenergic: An agent that produces stimulating adrenalin-like effects on the sympathetic nervous system.

allergen: A substance capable of causing an allergy or allergic reaction.

allergy: An antibody-antigen allergen reaction; hypersensitivity to a substance.

amphetamine: A stimulant to the central nervous system.

analgesic: A drug given to relieve pain without loss of consciousness.

analog (analogue): A substance structurally or chemically similar to another related drug or chemical for the purpose of changing the original drug's characteristics to produce an improved drug with fewer side effects or more therapeutic action.

anaphylaxis: An allergic hypersensitivity usually to a protein substance or drug; a severe, life-threatening allergic reaction accompanied by vasodilation, lowered blood pressure, and shock.

anesthetic: A drug that causes loss of sensation and insensibility to pain or touch.

antacid: A drug that neutralizes acidity, especially in the digestive tract.

antagonist: A drug that opposes a bodily system or expected effect.

antianaphylactic: Prevention of anaphylaxis. Often attained by administering repeated doses of a sensitizing substance too small to call an anaphylactic reaction; a way of desensitizing.

antianginal: A drug that relieves chest pain.

antianxiety drugs: Drugs used to relieve anxiety and emotional tension.

antiarrhythmic: A drug test prevents cardiac arrhythmias.

antibiotic: A drug used to kill living microorganisms, including gram-positive and gram-negative bacteria, that cause infection.

antibody: A protein substance which develops in response to and reacts with an invading antigen.

anticoagulant: A drug used to prevent blood clotting.

anticonvulsant: A drug that relieves or prevents convulsions.

antidiabetic: A drug that prevents or relieves diabetes.

antidiarrheal: A drug that relieves or corrects diarrhea.

antidote: Any substance that neutralizes or counteracts the effects of a poison.

antiemetic: A drug that prevents or relieves vomiting.

antifungal: A synthetic drug that destroys or inhibits fungal growth and yeast infections.

antigen: A foreign substance (virus, bacterium, or toxin) that induces the production of antibodies.

antihistamine: A drug used to treat and relieve allergy symptoms such as hay fever, and relieves symptoms of the common cold, urticaria, and pruritus.

anti-inflammatory: A drug used to treat and relieve pain, swelling, and tenderness.

antinauseant: A drug used to prevent or decrease nausea.

antipruritic: A drug, ointment, or solution that relieves itching.

antipsychotic: A drug used to treat schizophrenia, paranoia, and other psychotic disorders.

antipyretic: A drug given to reduce fever.

antiseptic: A topical drug used on living tissue which prevents or inhibits the growth of microorganisms, especially bacteria. (It does not necessarily kill them).

antispasmodic: A drug used to relieve or prevent muscular contractions, spasms, and convulsions.

antitussive: A drug given to relieve a cough.

antiviral: A drug used to combat viral infections and diseases.

aphrodisiac: A drug used to arouse or increase sexual desire.

astringent: A substance that produces shrinkage of mucous membranes or other tissues and decreases secretion.

bactericide: A substance that kills bacteria.

bacteriostatic: A substance that inhibits the growth of bacteria.

bore (synonymous with gauge): The inside diameter of a needle. Unlike the gauge, the bore is never assigned a specific number but is designated small or large.

buffered analgesic: A pill containing an antacid to reduce acidity.

butterfly needle: A specially designed needle of short length and high gauge. It has color-coded plastic tabs on each side to facilitate control of the needle during insertion. They are often used to start IVs on premature babies and geriatric patients with poor veins.

cancer: A tumor or unnatural growth in the body.

Candida: A genus of yeast-like fungi.

carcinogen: An agent that produces cancer.

carminative: An agent used to expel gas from the GI tract.

catalyst: A substance that increases the speed of a chemical reaction but is not used up nor permanently changed in any way by the reaction.

cathartic: A drug used to increase and hasten evacuation of the bowel (a laxative).

CD: An abbreviation for "continual dosing," usually part of the trade name (Cardizem CD).

chemotherapy: The use of chemical agents to treat or control a disease. It is used when cancer is disseminated, when it cannot be surgically removed, or when it fails to respond to radiation.

cholinergic: A type of receptor activated by the neurotransmitter acetylcholine.

cocaine: A CNS stimulant extracted from leaves of the Erythroxylan coca plant. It is a Schedule II drug used as a surface anesthesia of the ear, nose, throat, rectum, and vagina. Street names include blow, coke, flake, gold dust, rock, snow, and white girl. Cocaine combined with heroin is known as a speed ball.

contraindication: A symptom indicating inappropriateness of a drug or treatment. A specific factor physicians consider prior to selecting medication for an individual.

corticosteroid: A hormone produced by adrenal glands, or a topical or oral drug used to reduce inflammation and treat allergic rhinitis.

CR: An abbreviation for "controlled release," usually part of the trade name (Norpace CR).

decongestants: A drug used to symptomatically treat nasal congestion; constricts dilated arterioles reducing nasal blood flow and improving drainage.

dependence: A severe attachment to a drug or agent; an addiction.

depressant: A reduction in the activities of body parts.

depression: An unnatural state of lethargy, inactivity, and sadness.

desensitize: To lessen the sensitivity by administering an antigen.

diaphoretic: A drug used to induce and increase perspiration.

disinfectant (germicide): A chemical used on inanimate objects that kill or inhibit growth of microorganisms. It is used to sterilize instruments but not used on the human body.

diuretic: A drug used to increase the excretion of urine. It is used to treat edema and hypertension.

dose: A specified amount of medicinal preparation to be administered at one time.

drug of choice: A drug shown to be of particular clinical value in treating a specific diseased state. It is preferred above all other similar drugs because of its superior therapeutic results.

drug tolerance: A decreased susceptibility to the effects of a drug caused by continued use.

DS: An abbreviation for a double dosage (double-strength); usually part of the trade name (Bactrim DS).

emetic: A drug that stimulates vomiting.

emollient: A substance that softens the skin and soothes irritation.

enteric coating: This special coating allows pills to pass through the stomach and dissolve in the small intestine. This type of coating is used to minimize stomach irritation, but it also takes longer to absorb.

enzyme: A substance formed by living cells that promotes a particular chemical reaction in the body by functioning as a catalyst.

exacerbation: When the symptoms of a disease are most severe.

expectorant: A drug used to liquify mucus from the respiratory tract which increases secretions making it easier to expel mucus.

extended release: Slow dissolving; prolongs release of agent into the system.

gauge: The inside diameter of a needle. The smaller the number, the larger the diameter.

general anesthetic: An agent that eliminates pain and voluntary muscle control, then induces unconsciousness.

habit forming: The condition whereby drugs are routinely taken as a matter of course, not as a matter of necessity. Withdrawal symptoms are not seen on cessation of the habit. User becomes accustomed to frequent use.

half-life: The time required for drug levels in the serum to decrease from 100 percent to 50 percent. The half-life of a drug can be significantly prolonged with liver or kidney disease. For example, digoxin (Lanoxin) has a half-life of approximately 30 hours. Geriatric patients with poor liver and kidney functioning often develop levels of toxicity because circulating levels of the active drug remain high for long periods of time.

hematinic: An agent that tends to increase the hemoglobin content of the blood; usually contains iron.

histamine: An amino acid that produces the symptoms of allergic reactions.

hormone: An agent secreted by the endocrine glands that produces or alters bodily functions.

hypersensitivity: Excessive or abnormal sensitivity/susceptibility to the action of a given agent.

hypnotic: A drug used to produce sleep.

immunization: A process of inducing or providing immunity by administering an artificial immunizing agent. It is usually given in childhood to reduce the occurrence of vaccine-preventable diseases.

immunosuppressive: An agent that interferes with the body systems that resist infection and foreign materials.

infection: The process of a pathogenic agent invading the body, multiplying, and causing injury.

inhalation: The act of drawing air into the lungs by breathing; medication administration by means of a special apparatus such as an inhalator, vaporizer, atomizer, nebulizer, intermittent positive pressure machine, or respirator.

injection: The act of forcing liquid into a body part; medication is administered either directly into the bloodstream or tissue.

insulin syringe: A special syringe designed to measure only insulin. It is calibrated in units; all other syringes are calibrated in milliliters.

intrinsic factor: A substance in the gastric wall that is necessary for vitamin B12 absorption.

irrigation: The cleansing of a canal by flushing with water or other fluids; used in the washing of a wound.

LA: An abbreviation for long-acting. It is usually part of the trade name of sustained-release, long-acting drugs such as Entex LA.

laxative: A mild cathartic that loosens and promotes bowel movements without discomfort.

L-dopa: L is the abbreviation for levorotary, a term used to describe a drug's molecules which are arranged in a way that bends polarized light to the left.

lethal dose: The amount of a drug that will cause death.

loading dose: An amount that is generally twice the maintenance dose; given if the therapeutic effect of a drug is desired immediately to treat a medical crisis. This promptly raises the serum levels of the drug to the therapeutic range to initiate treatment. The loading dose is given only once, then maintenance doses are used for subsequent treatment.

local anesthesia: Introduction of a drug, usually injected, that temporarily eliminates pain by interfering with local nerve transmission, causing a deadening in a small, limited area.

long acting: See LA.

LSD: Lysergic acid diethylamide. Taken orally, it is frequently absorbed in a sugar cube. LSD is a Schedule I drug. Its street name is usually "acid."

maintenance dose: The standard dose prescribed by the physician. It is generally one-half the loading dose.

marijuana: The dried, flowering tops and leaves (and occasionally seeds and stems) of the Cannabis sativa plant. It is often hand-rolled into cigarettes and smoked; a Schedule I drug. (A synthetic variation has been approved as an antiemetic for cancer treatment.) Street names include Acapulco gold, grass, joint, Mary Jane, pot, and reefer.

maximal dose: The largest amount of drug given, still producing the desired effect.

metabolism: The chemical energy of foodstuffs transformed to mechanical energy or heat.

metastasis: The spread of cancer cells from one body part to another.

microorganism: An organism not visible to the naked eye that may or may not produce a disease.

minerals: Naturally occurring, inorganic substances necessary to body function.

minimal dose: See *therapeutic dose.*

miotic: A drug that causes the pupil to contract.

mydriatic: A drug that causes the pupil to dilate.

narcotic: A drug used to relieve pain and produce sleep or stupor.

needles: Slender, hollow instruments which are classified according to gauge and length and are used to inject liquids.

oral: Medication given by mouth.

oxytocic: A drug used to produce uterine contractions.

palliative: A drug which provides relief of symptoms but does not cure the disease.

parenteral: All methods of giving medications by means of a needle or cannula introduced through the skin, including sub-Q, IM, IV, intraspinal, intrasternal, intracapsular, and intraorbital.

pathogen: A microorganism capable of causing disease (virus, bacterium, or fungus).

PCP: Phencyclidene. It may come in a powder, tablet, or capsule form, or it can also be injected. Schedule I drug; no legal use in United States. Street names include angel dust, cosmos, jet, peace pill, super joint, and whack.

PDR: Physicians' Desk Reference.

peak levels: Measurements which indicate the highest serum level achieved following a single dose of a drug. They are used to determine if serum levels of a drug are high enough to produce a therapeutic effect or are too high, which would cause toxicity. Peak levels are determined by blood tests.

placebo: An inactive preparation commonly known as sugar pills. They are used in controlled pharmaceutical studies to determine effectiveness of a tested medication. In most situations, the patient is unaware he or she is being administered a placebo. It may be given in place of an actual drug to gratify the patient.

prophylactic: A drug used to prevent the development of a disease; includes vaccines, birth control pills, hormones, or vitamins.

prostaglandins: Short-acting hormones that perform many functions in the body and exert their effect close to the site of production.

prothrombin: A protein produced by the liver necessary for normal blood coagulation.

prothrombin time: A measurement of the prothrombin level in the blood. This measurement is performed routinely to assess the effectiveness of anticoagulant therapy.

SA: An abbreviation for sustained action. It is usually part of the trade name of sustained release, long-acting drugs, such as Choledyl SA.

sedative: A drug that exerts a quiet, relaxing effect; relieves anxiety without inducing sleep.

shock: A sudden drop in blood pressure due to injury or blood loss.

side effect: Any action or effect other than the desired effect.

SL: An abbreviation for sublingual. It is usually part of the trade name such as Isordil SL.

Spansules: A registered trademark of SmithKline pharmaceutical company, designating a slow-release capsule such as Compazine Spansules.

SR: An abbreviation for slow release or sustained release. It is usually part of the trade name, such as Theospan SR.

steroid: A compound which accelerates physical development by increasing body weight and muscular strength. It may be taken orally or injected directly into muscle. Street names include roids, juice, and d-ball.

stimulant: A drug that temporarily increases activity or hastens actions in the body or in an organ; counteracts depression.

sustained action: See *SA.*

sustained (slow) release: See *SR.*

therapeutic dose: The smallest amount of drug that will produce a desired effect.

therapeutic index: A measurement calculated during animal testing of any new drug. It reflects the relative margin of safety inherent between the dose needed to produce a therapeutic effect and the dose which produces toxic effects. The higher the therapeutic index the better, as it indicates the drug has a wide margin of safety. Penicillin has a therapeutic index of greater than 100. The therapeutic index of digoxin is less than 2. It is not uncommon for patients taking a therapeutic dose of digoxin to begin to exhibit symptoms of toxicity.

time release: See *extended release.*

titrate: The smallest dosage that will produce the desired effect for a specific individual.

tolerance: The capacity for enduring a large amount of a substance without exhibiting any adverse effects.

topical: Substances applied to the skin such as unguents, ointments, creams, sprays, emulsions, powders, liniments, or liquids.

toxic dose: Any dosage that causes a poisonous or potentially dangerous situation for the patient.

toxin: The poisonous substance released by microorganisms.

tranquilizer: A drug used to reduce anxiety without clouding consciousness; a sedative.

transdermal: Medication delivered through the skin by means of a patch.

trough levels: A measurement determined by a blood test indicating the lowest serum level of a drug which occurs just before the next dose is to be given.

vasopressor: A drug that produces vasoconstriction and an increase in blood pressure.

vial: A small glass bottle with a rubber stopper containing a liquid or powder for injection. The rubber stopper allows repeated doses of the drug to be withdrawn from the same vial.

withdrawal: Cessation of administration of a drug, especially a narcotic, to which a patient has become physically or psychologically addicted.

ABBREVIATIONS

In order for medications to be ordered, transcribed, and administered safely, health care employees must be thoroughly familiar with accepted standard abbreviations found in prescriptions and physician orders. Medical abbreviations are used internationally by both professional and nonprofessional personnel dealing with medications. Understanding the prescription abbreviations is critical and essential. Chapter 9 covers prescription slip requirements in detail.

Common Prescription Abbreviations

Abbreviation	Latin	Meaning
a.c.	ante cibum	before meals
AD	auris dextra	right ear
ad lib	ad libitum	as needed; at pleasure
alt hor	alternis horis	every other hour
amt		amount
ante		before
AS	auris sinistra	left ear
AU	auris utraque	both ears
b.i.d.	bis in die	twice a day
c̄	cum	with
C&S		culture and sensitivity
caps		capsules
d/c; D/C; DC; disc		discontinue
dil		dilute
disp		dispense
DSD		double starting dose
elix		elixir
et		and
ext		extract
FOB		foot of bed
fl oz		fluid ounce
g		gram
gr		grain
gtt	guttae	drops
h (hr)		hour
h.s.	hora somni	at bedtime; hour of sleep
I&O		intake and output
IM		intramuscular
IU		immunizing unit
IV		intravenous
L/min		liters per minute
mcg (μ)		micrograms
mEq		milliequivalent
noc; noct		at night
n.p.o.	nihil per os	nothing by mouth
occ.		occasionally
OD	oculus dexter	right eye
os		mouth
OS	oculus sinister	left eye
OTC		over the counter
OU	oculus uterque	both eyes
p̄	post	after

Abbreviation	Latin	Meaning
p.c.	post cibum	after meals
p.o.	per os	by mouth
p.r.n.	pro re nata	as needed
q	quaque	every
q2h	quaque 2 hora	every 2 hours
q4h	quaque 4 hora	every 4 hours
qd	quaque die	every day
qh	quaque hora	every hour
q.h.s.	quaque hora somni	every bedtime
q.i.d.	quater in die	four times per day
q.o.d.	quaque otra die	every other day
q.o.h.	quaque otra hora	every other hour
q.s.	quantum sufficit	quantity sufficient
Rx	symbol for recipe	prescription
ss	semis	one-half
s̄	sine	without
Sig.	signa	label; give directions on prescription
sl		sublingually
sol		solution
s.o.s.	si opus sit	if necessary or required
SSE		soap suds enema
stat	statim	immediately
sub-Q; subcu; subq		subcutaneous
tabs		tablet
t.i.d.	ter in die	three times per day
tinc		tincture
TKO		to keep open
T.O.		telephone order
top		topically
ung		ointment
vag		vaginally
V.O.		verbal order

You will find an inclusive list of commonly used abbreviations and symbols in Appendix A.

CHAPTER REVIEW

In most situations, reference material will be available to you. However, by being familiar with the medical terminology and specific medical elements (roots, prefixes, and suffixes) you should be able to define the following medical words.

1. analgesic _____

_____

_____

_____

_____

2. antacid _____

_____

_____

_____

_____

3. antiarrhythmic _____

_____

_____

_____

_____

4. antibody _____

_____

_____

_____

_____

5. anticoagulant _____

_____

_____

_____

_____

6. antidiarrheal _____

_____

_____

_____

_____

7. antipyretic _____

_____

_____

_____

_____

8. contraindication _____

_____

_____

_____

_____

9. decongestant _____

_____

_____

_____

_____

10. disinfectant _____

_____

_____

_____

_____

11. emetic _____

_____

_____

_____

_____

12. exacerbation _____

_____

_____

_____

_____

13. hypnotic _____

_____

_____

_____

_____

14. metabolism _____

_____

_____

_____

_____

15. parenteral _____

_____

_____

_____

_____

16. sedative _____

_____

_____

_____

_____

17. side effect _____

_____

_____

_____

_____

18. stimulant _____

_____

_____

_____

_____

19. topical _____

_____

_____

_____

_____

20. transdermal _____

_____

_____

_____

_____

21. Match the following abbreviations with the correct number of the definition.

____ a.	q.o.d.	1. at bedtime		16.	every other day
____ b.	Rx	2. as needed		17.	with
____ c.	stat	3. three times a day		18.	without
____ d.	ung	4. right eye		19.	over the counter
____ e.	p.r.n.	5. left eye		20.	immediately
____ f.	c̄	6. right ear		21.	ointment
____ g.	OS	7. left ear		22.	lotion
____ h.	OTC	8. both eyes		23.	every two hours
____ i.	p.c.	9. both ears		24.	by mouth
____ j.	b.i.d.	10. twice a day		25.	every four hours
____ k.	AS	11. four times a day			
____ l.	a.c.	12. after meals			
____ m.	h.s.	13. before meals			
____ n.	t.i.d.	14. on the counter			
____ o.	p.o.	15. prescription			

7

Measurements and Dosage Calculations

COMPETENCIES

At the end of this chapter, the student should be able to:

1. Read and write decimals correctly.
2. Read and write roman numerals correctly.
3. Provide the apothecary unit abbreviations.
4. Explain the importance of understanding both household and apothecaries' measurements.
5. Demonstrate proper usage of apothecary and metric system punctuation rules.
6. Name the three basic units of measurements in the metric system.
7. Provide the abbreviations of the household measurements.
8. Provide metric unit abbreviations.
9. Convert quantities in metric units to apothecary units.
10. Convert quantities in apothecary units to metric units.
11. Provide standard abbreviation for milliequivalent.
12. Determine approximate equivalents between apothecaries' and household measurements.

CHAPTER CONTENT

Measurements
Roman Numerals
  Roman Numeral Rules
Apothecary System
Abbreviations
Metric System
  Conversions Between Systems
  Meter
  Metric and Household Punctuation Rules
  Gram
  Liter

INTRODUCTION

A registered pharmacist has the responsibility to accurately calculate and prepare drugs and dosages for administration. Often the physician's assistant, nurse, or medical assistant has the responsibility to administer the prepared drug. Medical transcriptionists or secretaries transcribing drug orders may need to know how to calculate conversions. In order to perform this task effectively, a strong foundation of basic math is necessary for conversions and calculations.

The calculations explained and provided in this chapter are fairly basic; however, refer to supplemental math textbooks for additional reference if needed. Although .5 and 0.5 are the same figures, a misinterpretation could result in a 10-fold medication error. The correct placement of zeros and decimal points is crucial. By following basic punctuation rules, you can minimize problems for yourself, the physician, the patients, and other medical personnel.

MEASUREMENTS

Throughout the years there have been three systems of measurement—the apothecaries', metric, and household systems. Conversions between these systems are *approximations,* close but not exact.

ROMAN NUMERALS

We are accustomed to using arabic numerals in everyday calculations. They include numbers 0 through 9 and any combination of these. Roman numerals, which make use of letters to represent numeric values, are a part of the apothecaries' system of measurement. Roman numerals are often used when physicians write prescription orders or medication orders. Refer to Table 7-1 for roman numeral equivalents.

Roman Numeral Rules

The following steps assist you with reading and writing roman numerals.

1. When two roman numerals of the same value are repeated in sequence, you add their values. The same roman numeral may not be repeated more than three times.

    Example: III $(1 + 1 + 1) = 3$ XXX $(10 + 10 + 10) = 30$

2. When a roman numeral of a larger value is followed by one of a lesser value, add the values.

    Example: VI $= (5 + 1) = 6$ XII $= (10 + 2) = 12$

TABLE 7-1 ROMAN NUMERAL EQUIVALENTS

Arabic	Roman	Arabic	Roman
1	I	15	XV
2	II	20	XX
3	III	25	XXV
4	IV	30	XXX
5	V	40	XL
6	VI	50	L
7	VII	100	C
8	VIII	500	D
9	IX	1000	M
10	X		

3. A roman numeral of a lesser value followed by one of a larger value is subtracted from the larger value.

$$\text{Example: IX} = (10 - 1) = 9$$

4. A roman numeral placed between two numerals of a larger value is subtracted from the following numeral.

$$\text{Example: XIX} = 10 + (10 - 1) = 19 \qquad \text{XIV} = 10 + (5 - 1) = 14$$

5. Roman numerals over 100 are seldom used in medicine but have been provided in Table 7-1 for your information.

APOTHECARY SYSTEM

The *apothecary system,* which was once widely used by pharmacists in preparing prescriptions, has been replaced by the metric system. Although the apothecaries' system consists of roman numerals and common fractions, arabic numbers are most often used. The apothecaries' measurements divided the pound into 12 ounces, the ounce into 8 drams (480 grains), the dram into 3 scruples, and the scruple into 20 grains. (*Note:* The apothecaries' system divides the pound into 12 ounces whereas the household system divides the pound into 16 ounces.) The apothecaries' measurements you still see used for medications include grains (gr), drams (dr or the symbol ʒ) and ounce (oz or the symbol ℥). The grain was the most common apothecaries' unit, and is the smallest unit of weight used in the United States. It is based on the average weight of one grain of wheat. The two most widely used medications dispensed using grains were aspirin and morphine; however, recently these have been converted to milligrams, probably to prevent any confusion with the gram.

Apothecaries' measurements are also used as household measures, primarily liquid volume. Examples include the pint, quart, and gallon. Other than the grain, the apothecaries' system of measurement is rarely used in pharmacology today. This system does not provide an equivalence for measuring length.

Depending on the medication being dispensed, occasionally household measurements are applied. Although these measurements tend to be less accurate, they are used more commonly than the apothecaries' or metric system for standard over-the-counter drugs such as antitussives (cough medicines), antacids, enemas, eye drops, and nasal drops. Measurements using a teaspoon, tablespoon, or dropper tend to be very subjective. What could be measured as one drop to one person might be three drops to the next individual. Spoon sizes also vary in size. Household measurements are frequently used when exact precision is not critical as they do not provide accurate measurements.

ABBREVIATIONS

Refer to Tables 7-2 and 7-3 for apothecaries' and household abbreviations. To reiterate, there are abbreviations used in pharmacology that may not be appropriate in medical transcription.

METRIC SYSTEM

The French Academy of Sciences created the *metric system* in 1790. The United States showed little interest in this system, and it was not actually made legal by Congress in the states until 1866. It was not until 1968

TABLE 7-2 APOTHECARIES' WEIGHT AND VOLUME ABBREVIATIONS

gr = grains
dr or ʒ = dram/teaspoon
oz or ʒ = ounce
fl oz = fluid ounce
pt = pint
qt = quart
gal = gallon
lb/# = pound

TABLE 7-3 HOUSEHOLD ABBREVIATIONS

gtt = drops
tsp/t = teaspoon
tbsp/T = tablespoon
c = cup
pt = pint
qt = quart
gal = gallon

Congress authorized a 3-year study of metric conversion. As a result of this study, it was determined a 10-year, step-by-step conversion to the metric system would be instituted. Although strictly voluntary, it was felt this conversion program would promote the increased use of metric units of measurement by business and industry. In 1988, the metric system, officially known as the International System of Units (SI), was adopted as the exclusive unit of measurement by the American Medical Association. SI is used for the following measurements: meters measure length, grams measure weight and solids, liters measure volume and fluids, and square meters measure surface. The focus in this chapter is on length, weight, and volume.

Conversions Between Systems

Lay people need know only a few metric units to get through an average day. Although the metric system is the only system being taught in the health care field, it is not yet used exclusively. Until it is, conversions between systems must be made. Physicians and medical professionals calculate conversions daily. For example, medications ordered in drams or ounces (apothecaries'), are manufactured and labeled using the metric system. The medical transcriptionist and medical secretary will often transcribe medical and doctors' orders, and may restock supply rooms. Although the medical secretary will not perform the actual drug or dosage calculations, it is vital he or she understands how to convert from one system to another, and be able to detect errors in basic calculations.

Keep in mind, most conversions are approximate rather than exact equivalents.

The fundamental unit of length in the metric system is the *meter*, from which all units of length in this system are derived. Metric prefixes, added to most metric units to increase or decrease their size, denote the size of a metric unit. Each prefix is based on multiples of 10. For example, the prefix "centi" means one-hundredth; therefore, 1 cm = 1 one-hundredth of a meter. Prefixes are written in lowercase letters—centi, milli, deci, and so on. The three units you will see most often are the meter (m), centimeter (cm), and millimeter (mm). Refer to Table 7-4 for the seven most common metric prefixes.

TABLE 7-4   METER = LENGTH

Metric Prefix	Metric Measurement	Abbrev.	Meters
kilo-	kilometer	km	1,000 meters
hect-	hectometer	hm	100
deka- (deca-)	dekameter	dam	10
meter	meter	m	1
deci-	decimeter	dm	0.1 of a meter
centi-	centimeter	cm	0.01 of a meter
milli-	millimeter	mm	0.001 of a meter

Meter

To compare common metric measurements to household measurements, the meter is equal to 39.37 inches (slightly longer than 1 yard); 2½ centimeters are approximately 1 inch; and a decimeter is roughly 4 inches.

Metric and Household Punctuation Rules

Punctuation rules are covered in detail in chapter 8; however, for clarification, a few basic punctuation and notation rules are given in this chapter.

1. Metric measurements are generally abbreviated, but are not punctuated unless at the end of a sentence. The same abbreviation is used for the singular and plural forms. Do not abbreviate nonmetric units of measurements. There is one space between the number and the unit.

    Examples: 5 g   20 ounces   4 cm   10 ml   3 feet   15 mg

2. The recent trend is to move away from roman numerals. However, you will see some used in the dispensing and recording of medications. In the apothecaries' system, the unit or abbreviation is usually expressed in lowercase roman numerals and the measurement comes before the number.

    Examples: gr ii   gr x or gr 10   gr xx or gr 20

3. Quantities less than 1 are expressed as fractions *except* ½. In the writing of prescriptions you will find one-half is often expressed by the symbol *ss*.

    Examples: ¼ grains = gr ¼
    1½ grains = gr iss
    three ounces = oz iii
    ½ grains = gr ss

4. The metric and English unit or abbreviation always follows the amount. Always use standard abbreviations and skip one space between the number and the unit.

    Examples: 10 g   15 ml   18 cm   42 L

5. Decimals are used for fractional units rather than fractions.

    Examples: 1.4 ml   3.5 g   8.9 cm

6. Unnecessary zeros after a decimal point are omitted.

    Examples: 4.5 g not 4.50 g   8.75 ml not 8.750 ml

7. Zeros are used to emphasize the decimal point for fractional units less than 1 to prevent confusion and potential dosage errors.

    Examples: 0.25 mg   0.5 ml   0.125 mg

Conversion between units of length in the metric system involves moving the decimal point to the right or to the left. To calculate movement of the decimal, list the units in order from largest to smallest. This will indicate how many places to move the decimal point and in which direction.

Example 1: To convert 5100 dm to m, move the decimal point the same number of places in the same direction.

$$\text{km} \quad \text{hm} \quad \text{dam} \quad \overset{\frown}{\text{m}} \quad \text{dm} \quad \text{cm} \quad \text{mm}$$

one position to the left

5100 dm = 510 m

Example 2: To convert 0.45 m to cm, again, move the decimal point the same number of places in the same direction.

$$\text{km} \quad \text{hm} \quad \text{dam} \quad \overset{\frown}{\text{m}} \quad \text{dm} \quad \text{cm} \quad \text{mm}$$

two positions to the right

0.45 m = 45 cm

Exercise 1: Convert 61.5 cm to m.

$$\text{km} \quad \text{hm} \quad \text{dam} \quad \text{m} \quad \text{dm} \quad \text{cm} \quad \text{mm}$$

_____ positions to the _____

61.5 cm = _____ m

Exercise 2: Convert 6501 m to km.

$$\text{km} \quad \text{hm} \quad \text{dam} \quad \text{m} \quad \text{dm} \quad \text{cm} \quad \text{mm}$$

_____ positions to the _____

6501 m = _____ km

Exercise 3: Convert 55 mm to cm.

$$\text{km} \quad \text{hm} \quad \text{dam} \quad \text{m} \quad \text{dm} \quad \text{cm} \quad \text{mm}$$

_____ positions to the _____

55 mm = _____ cm

Kilometers are often used by runners to measure distance. To convert kilometers to miles, multiply by 0.62. To convert miles to kilometers, divide by 0.62.

Gram

The basic unit of weight (mass) in the metric system is the *gram* (g). The gram is a very small unit of mass; 1 gram can be compared to the weight of a paperclip. The same prefixes used to measure length are used to measure weight. The three weight measurements most often used are the gram (g), milligram (mg), and the kilogram (kg). The microgram has been added to the weight category. The prefix micro- refers to one-millionth or .000001. You will see this used in some drug calculations. It is commonly abbreviated mcg (μg).

The conversion of moving the decimal point to the right or left is also the same as previously shown for length.

Example 1: Converting 510 g to hg requires moving the decimal point the same number of places in the same direction.

$$\text{kg} \quad \overset{\frown}{\text{hg}} \quad \text{dag} \quad \text{g} \quad \text{dg} \quad \text{cg} \quad \text{mg}$$

Two positions to the left

510 g = 5.10 hg

Two places to the left

TABLE 7-5   GRAM = MASS AND/OR WEIGHT

Metric Prefix	Metric Measurement	Abbrev.
kilo-	kilogram	kg
hect-	hectogram	hg
deka- (deca-)	dekagram	dag
meter	gram	g
deci-	decigram	dg
centi-	centigram	cg
milli-	milligram	mg
micro-	microgram	mcg (μg)

Exercise 1:   Convert 4.93 dag to cg.

kg   hg   dag   g   dg   cg   mg
_____ positions to the _____
4.93 dag = _____ cg

Exercise 2:   Convert 6 cg to g.

kg   hg   dag   g   dg   cg   mg
_____ positions to the _____
6 cg = _____ g

Exercise 3:   Convert 38.1 mg to g.

kg   hg   dag   g   dg   cg   mg
_____ positions to the _____
38.1 mg = _____ g

Exercise 4:   A doctor recommends a patient take 3.5 g of vitamin C per week. What is the daily dosage in milligrams?

A few basic weight conversions are provided in Table 7-6.

The physician often records newborn and infant weights using grams. Laypeople are not accustomed to hearing weights in grams. To convert grams into an apothecaries' weight readily understood, a conversion formula is necessary. Using Table 7-5, complete the following exercises using the example provided.

Example 1:   The newborn weighed 4400 grams. Convert to pounds.

We know 2.2 lb = 1000 g, therefore:

$$\frac{4400 \times 2.2}{1000} = \frac{9680}{1000} = 9.68 \text{ lb}$$

Exercise 1:   In the last 3 months, the baby gained 740 g. Convert to pounds.

TABLE 7-6   APPROXIMATE METRIC WEIGHT EQUIVALENTS

Metric		Equivalent	Metric		Equivalent
1000 mcg	=	1 mg	0.3 g	=	gr 5
1 mg	=	gr 1/60	0.5 g	=	gr 7½
5 mg	=	gr 1/12	0.6 g	=	gr 10
10 mg	=	gr 1/6	1 g	=	gr 15
15 mg	=	gr 1/4	2 g	=	gr 30
20 mg	=	gr 1/3	3 g	=	gr 45
25 mg	=	gr 3/8	4 g	=	dr i or ℨ i
30 mg	=	gr 1/2	5 g	=	gr 75
40 mg	=	gr 2/3	6 g	=	gr 90
50 mg	=	gr 3/4	7½ g	=	dr 2
60 mg	=	gr i	10 g	=	dr 2½
75 mg	=	gr i 1/4	15 g	=	dr 4
1000 mg	=	1 g	30 g	=	oz i or ℥ i; gr 480
0.1 g	=	gr 1½	360 g	=	12 oz
0.2 g	=	gr 3	500 g	=	1.1 lb
0.25 g	=	gr 4	1000 g (1 kg)	=	2.2 lb

Exercise 2:   The patient was instructed to take gr X Tylenol. How many mg is that? _____

_____

_____

_____

Exercise 3:   The physician orders the patient to take 900 mg daily; each tablet contains gr v. How many tablets must the patient take? _____

_____

_____

_____

Exercise 4:   Mom is concerned her child is losing weight. The physician's progress notes indicate the last office weight was 9650 g. Mom states baby now weighs 16 lb. Has the baby gained or lost weight? How much weight? _____

_____

_____

_____

Liter

The basic unit of volume (fluid or liquid) in the metric system is the *liter* (L/l). The volume refers to how much a container can hold. There is a slight difference between dry and liquid measurements. For our calculations, we will use only liquid measures. One liter is defined as the volume of a 10 cm square box.

One cubic centimeter ($cm^3 = 1$ cc) is another common way of expressing 1 ml. One cc is the amount of space occupied by 1 ml of liquid. Just as with the units of length and mass, the units of volume utilize the same metric prefixes. The two volume measures you will use most often are the liter (L) and the milliliter (ml or mL) (see Table 7-7).

The process of conversion between these units is also the same as length and weight.

Example 1: Converting 187 ml to liters requires moving the decimal the same number of places in the same direction.

kl   hl   dal   L   dl   cl   ml

Three positions to the left

1 8 7 ml = 0.187 L

Example 2: Convert 5 L 34 ml to liters.

kl   hl   dal   L   dl   cl   ml

Three positions to the left

.0 3 4 ml = .034 L

5 L 34 ml = 5 L + .034 L

= 5.034 L

Tables 7-8 and 7-9 may be useful in solving the next set of exercises. Show all your work for the following:

Exercise 1: Convert 4.67 L to cc. _____

_____

_____

_____

_____

TABLE 7-7   LITER = VOLUME

Metric Prefix	Metric Measurement	Abbrev.	Liters
kilo-	kiloliter	kl	1,000 liters
hect-	hectoliter	hl	100
deka- (deca-)	dekaliter	dal	10
meter	liter	L	1
deci-	deciliter	dl	0.1 of a liter
centi-	centiliter	cl	0.01 of a liter
milli-	milliliter	ml	0.001 of a liter

TABLE 7-8 APPROXIMATE METRIC EQUIVALENTS FOR VOLUME

Metric	Apothecaries'	Household
0.06 ml	1 minim	1 gtt
0.5 ml	8 minims	
1 ml = 1 cc	no equivalent	15 gtt
4 ml = 4 cc	1 fl dr	almost 1 tsp
5 ml = 5 cc	1¼ fl dr	1 tsp
15 ml	4 fl dr	1 tbsp (3 tsp)
30 ml = 30 cc	8 fl dr = 1 fl oz	2 tbsp
50 ml	1¾ fl oz	
250 ml	8 fl oz	1 c
500 ml	1 pt = 16 fl oz	1 pt
1000 ml = 1 L	1 qt = 32 fl oz	1 qt
4000 ml	1 gal = 4 qt	1 gal

Exercise 2: Oxygen constitutes 19 percent of atmospheric air. How much O2 is in 50 L of air? _____

_____

_____

_____

_____

Exercise 3: Your physician purchases 12 L of flu vaccine. Each injection is 3 cm³. How many patients can be immunized? _____

_____

_____

_____

_____

TABLE 7-9 APPROXIMATE METRIC EQUIVALENTS FOR DRY MEASUREMENTS

Metric (dry)	Apothecaries	Household
60 mg	gr 1	
0.5 g	gr 7½	⅛ tsp
1 g	gr 15	¼ tsp
4 g	gr 60 = 1 dram	1 tsp
15 g	dr 4	1 tbsp
30 g	1 oz	2 tbsp

Exercise 4: The drugstore where you work purchases one 5 L bulk container of cough syrup. You repackage the cough syrup into 250 ml bottles. How many bottles can you fill? _____

_____

_____

_____

More than 90 percent of the world's population utilize the metric system of measurement. It is essential to be able to convert from U.S. customary units to metric units. It may be necessary to convert a patient's weight or height between systems. Conversions most frequently seen are those converting meters or centimeters into yards, feet, or inches. Convert between units using the conversion factor. Multiply to change a larger unit to a smaller unit; divide to change a smaller unit to a larger unit. Keep in mind that these are approximate equivalents.

Example 1: Convert 100 yd to meters.

1 meter = 1.09 yards

The conversion factor is 1.09.

You are converting to a larger unit. Divide by the conversion factor.

$100 \div 1.09 = 91.7$ meters

Another way to do this is: 1 yard = 0.91 meters;

100 yards = 0.91 ($\times$ 100) = 91 meters.

Example 2: 1 c = ? ml

1 c = 8 fl oz

30 ml = 1 fl oz

The conversion factor is 30.

You are converting to a smaller unit. Multiply by the conversion factor.

$30 \times 8 = 240$ ml

1 c = 240 ml

TABLE 7-10

Units of Length	Units of Weight	Units of Volume
1 m = 3.28 ft	28.35 g = 1 oz	1 L = 1.06 qt
1 cm = .39 in	454 g = 1 lb	1 ml = 15 gtt
1.61 km = 1 mile	1 kg = 2.2 lb	15 ml = 1 tbsp
0.91 m = 1 yd	0.454 kg = 1 lb	30 ml = 1 fl oz
0.305 m = 1 ft	30 g = 1 oz	1 pt = 0.473 L
2.54 cm = 1 in	500 g = 1.1 lb	1 qt = 0.946 L
1 m = 1.09 yd		8 fl oz = 1 c

Exercise 1: You have 1 cup of liquid Tylenol. Your child is to take 15 ml four times per day. How many days will 1 cup last? _____

_____

_____

_____

Exercise 2: Your patient states he runs 12 miles q.o.d. Is it likely he could finish a 15 km race? Make the conversion. _____

_____

_____

_____

Exercise 3: Convert a toddler's weight of 8.8 kg to lb. _____

_____

_____

_____

Exercise 4: The physician suggests you walk 1/2 mile per day. Convert this to km. _____

_____

_____

_____

MILLIEQUIVALENT/UNIT

There are two other measurements used in prescribing medications. The *milliequivalent* (mEq) and the *unit* (U). The milliequivalent is one-thousandth (1/1000) of an equivalent weight of a chemical. The "unit" is a standardized amount needed to produce a *desired effect*. You will see "units" used with penicillin, insulin, and heparin. The term unit varies for each drug measured. Arabic numbers are used with the corresponding abbreviation.

Examples: 20 mEq   5000 U

MEASURING TEMPERATURE

Finally, the two common scales used to measure temperature are the *Fahrenheit* (F) and *centigrade* (C) scales. Patients are accustomed to thermometers that measure the average temperature at 98.6, which is the Fahrenheit measurement. Because many clinical thermometers use the centigrade scale, health care employees performing patient care must be able to convert from one scale to the other. If you are responsible for taking patient vitals, you should be familiar with the formulas for converting from one system to the other. As this does not fall into the realm of a medical secretary or a medical transcriptionist, it is not covered in this text.

Measurement and Dosage Punctuation Rules

COMPETENCIES

At the end of this chapter, the student should be able to:

1. Explain why the use of proper punctuation is essential.
2. Demonstrate proper usage of punctuation rules.
3. Explain when arabic numbers are used.
4. Explain when roman numerals are used.
5. Demonstrate accuracy when keying or writing measurements or dosages containing numbers, abbreviations, and symbols.

CHAPTER CONTENTS

Measurement and Dosage Punctuation Rules to Follow

INTRODUCTION

Accuracy in documenting medication dosages and frequencies is essential. To reiterate from chapter 7, the medical assistant may be responsible for administering medications. The medical secretary, as part of the daily routine, may be transcribing physician's orders or dictation, ordering and reordering medications, verifying prescription labels, answering calls from other physicians' offices and patients, and so on. Office personnel must have a thorough understanding of punctuation rules, know standard measurement and dosage abbreviations, and know when abbreviations can and cannot be used.

To avoid critical errors, medical professionals must be technically proficient with pharmacology punctuation.

As stressed in previous chapters, use of proper punctuation is essential when dealing with medications to prevent or minimize medication administration errors. As a reminder, metric measurements are generally abbreviated but not punctuated. The same abbreviation is used for the singular and plural forms. Except at the end of the sentence, there are no periods used in these abbreviations. English measurements are generally written out unless used in a table. However, measurements used in conjunction with medications are often abbreviated, such as teaspoon, tablespoon, ounces, and pounds.

MEASUREMENT AND DOSAGE PUNCTUATION RULES TO FOLLOW

1. There is one space between the arabic number and the metric or household unit.

   Examples: 5 g   20 ounces   4 cm
   10 ml   3 feet   15 mg

2. As a rule, do not punctuate uppercase abbreviations.

   Examples: BUN   PKU   CBC   PERRLA

3. Do not punctuate scientific abbreviations keyed in mixed case letters.

   Examples: Rx   mEq   Rh   Na   pH

4. In the apothecaries' system, the measurement *usually* comes before the number. Occasionally, roman numerals are used. Refer to chapter 7 and to medical transcription guidelines for clarity on roman numeral rules. Roman numerals I to III are handwritten with dots above a solid line for clarity.

   Examples: gr X   tsp 2   iï

5. With the centigrade or Fahrenheit symbol for degrees "°," do not leave a space between the number and the unit. Capitalize the C and the F.

   Examples: 25°C   98°F

6. To ensure accuracy, for a number less than one, place a zero before the decimal point to call attention to it and to prevent interpretation errors.

   Examples: 0.25 mg   0.5 g

7. Use commas to group numbers in units of three or more; however, omit commas in four digit figures.

   Examples: 100,000 wbc's   (or 100,000 wbc)
   1500 ml $4300   25,860

8. When a specific number is used with the "every hour" abbreviation, no periods or spaces are used. This may differ from rules given for a medical transcriptionist.

   Examples: q4h   q6h

9. A colon is used between hours and minutes indicating the time of day.

   Examples: 8:30 a.m.   10:15 p.m.
   4 p.m. but not 4:00 p.m.

Colons are **not** used when expressing military time.

Examples: 1800 hours   1630 hours

10. Capitalize trade names, brand name drugs, and trademarked materials. Do not capitalize generic names.

Examples: Tevdek   Steri-Strips   gentamicin

11. Capitalize the name of a genus but not the name of the species that follows it.

Examples: Escherichia coli (E. coli)
Mycobacterium tuberculosis (M. tuberculosis)

12. Measurements including lab values, medication dosages, BP, TPR, size, weight, and age are expressed in figures rather than in words.

Examples: The patient was 27 years of age.
He was discharged on Lanoxin 0.25 mg.
Take Diabinese, 1 tablet daily.

13. Use figures to express numbers containing decimals.

Examples: His direct bilirubin was 0.5 mg.
Her knee was injected with 0.5% Xylocaine.

14. Use figures when numbers are used directly with symbols, words, or abbreviations. Do not space between the number and symbol.

Examples: 2+ edema   50%   #8 Foley   15 mg b.i.d.

15. Always use decimal points rather than fractions with metric measurements, even when dictated as fractions.

Examples: 12.5 g   2.5 cm   15.25 mg   8.25 km

16. Use numerals for fractional measurements preceding a noun. Use a hyphen to join the fraction to the unit of measurement. This rule may differ from that of medical transcriptionists.

Examples: 3/4-pound tumor   1/4-inch long   1½-inch scar

CHAPTER REVIEW

A. Correctly rewrite the following:

1. Take fifteen milligrams two times daily. _____

_____

_____

_____

_____

2. The prescription was written for Lanoxin point twenty-five milligrams. _____

_____

_____

_____

_____

3. escherichia coli _____

_____

_____

_____

4. Temperature on admission was ninety-nine point seven degrees Fahrenheit. _____

_____

_____

_____

5. The medication is to be taken every four hours. _____

_____

_____

_____

B. Circle the correct answer.

6. 5 g   5g
7. 10 oz   10 oz.
8. 15ml   15 ml
9. 24 #   24#
10. 99° F   99°F

C. Write the abbreviations for the following:

11. _____ milliequivalent
12. _____ liter
13. _____ prescription
14. _____ grams
15. _____ grain

Understanding Prescription Slips and Prescription Labels

COMPETENCIES

At the end of this chapter, the student should be able to:

1. List all items that must be included on an ambulatory care prescription slip.
2. Explain who may write a prescription.
3. Describe the parts of a prescription slip.
4. Explain why prescription pads should be safely secured.
5. List the steps for safeguarding a prescription pad.
6. Explain the clerical steps for refilling a patient's prescription.
7. Accurately define prescription abbreviations.
8. Name two classifications of medications having an automatic stop policy.

CHAPTER CONTENT

Prescription Medications versus Over-the-Counter Drugs
Prescription Slip Content
Prescription Labels
Over-the-Counter Labels
Refilling Prescriptions
Clerical Steps for Refilling a Prescription

INTRODUCTION

In a medical setting, the physician determines which medications to prescribe. In order to have a prescription filled, laws require detailed information from the physician or dentist. The medical assistant, medical secretary, or medical receptionist in an ambulatory care setting may need to verify prescriptions written with the pharmacy filling the order. Although the format of prescription slips in an acute care setting and a doctor's office are different, the information required is basically the same. This chapter focuses on the ambulatory care setting and specific requirements for having a prescription filled.

PRESCRIPTION MEDICATIONS VERSUS OVER-THE-COUNTER DRUGS

Medicines are divided into two categories: prescription medications requiring a licensed clinical physician's or dentist's order and (2) over-the-counter (OTC) medicines which do not require a physician's order.

The physician has a professional obligation to the patient to determine the appropriate drug or product to prescribe.

A *prescription,* Latin for "a written order," is a written legal document with all the necessary information needed by the pharmacist and the patient. All prescription slips follow a specific format and most are preprinted on 5½" × 4¼" pads with the physician's name, the physician's office name, address, and telephone number. Occasionally the DEA narcotic number may be printed on the slip also as discussed in step 7 on the following pages (see Figure 9-1).

PRESCRIPTION SLIP CONTENT

This chapter primarily focuses on the prescription slip procedures in the ambulatory care setting.

R.F. HUTTEL, M.D. & ASSOCIATES, LTD.
5015 Shady Lane
Nowhere, State USA

| OFFICE PHONE | BUSINESS OFFICE |
| 555-8158 | 555-4147 |

Rx   DEA# AS2171996

Pt's Name _____

Pt's Address _____ Date _____

Label
Refills 0 - 1 - 2 - p.r.n.
Physician Reg. No. _____

_____M.D._____M.D.
Dispense as Written   Substitution Permitted

FIGURE 9-1 Physician's Office Prescription Slip

A prescription (Rx) slip includes the following:

1. *Patient's name and address.* The address is required when a prescription is filled for an outpatient.
2. *Date.* The date the prescription is written.
3. *Drug name.* Generic or trade—the chemical name is usually not used.
4. *Subscription.* The physician should indicate specific directions for the pharmacist such as route of administration, the total number of tablets or capsules to dispense, the dosage and frequency, the length of treatment, and/or the number of refills permitted. (Realistically, usually only the medication, dosage, form, and number of tablets or capsules are indicated. The amount of medication prescribed should be recorded in longhand as well as in numeric form to prevent it from being altered.
5. *Signa/Sig* (Latin for label). Gives instructions to the patient, such as what drug to take, how much, and how often (refer back to step 4).
6. *Signature line.* There is a preprinted line(s) on the bottom of the slips, followed by "M.D." (Occasionally slips will include a space for either DAW (dispense as written) or substitution signature lines). In order to be valid, the prescription slip must be signed by the physician with nonerasable ink.
7. *Drug Enforcement Administration* (DEA) Registration Number. The physician's registration number is required for controlled substances (see chapter 2 for controlled substance information). Now many third party payers also require a registration number prior to payment. If the number is not preprinted, it must be recorded for all narcotics prescribed.

Some medications, such as antibiotics and narcotics, have an automatic stop policy. A new physician's order must be secured before a refill may be obtained.

All prescription pads should be maintained by the physician or dentist in a secure location; however, it is the responsibility of all medical office personnel to prevent the misuse (stealing or forging) of prescription pads and slips. Prescription slips are legal documents used to control the legal sale of drugs and to ensure drugs are prescribed safely and effectively, under close supervision of a licensed physician or dentist. The actual hard copy of the prescription slip must be retained for a minimum of 7 years as determined by the physician's office policy. Figure 9-2 illustrates a sample prescription slip filled out by a physician. Refer to state guidelines for any questions on prescription slip retention.

PRESCRIPTION LABELS

Once a prescription is filled, the information on the drug label (Figure 9-3) is essential in helping the patient understand how and when to administer the medication. The label provides the following information:

R.F. HUTTEL, M.D. & ASSOCIATES, LTD.
5015 Shady Lane
Nowhere, State USA

OFFICE PHONE
555-8158

BUSINESS OFFICE
555-4147

℞

DEA# AS2171996

Pt's Name _Deborah Reinier_

Pt's Address _____ Date _____

Lanoxin 0.125
ⅰ qd p.o.

Label
Refills 0 - 1 - 2 (p.r.n.)

Physician Reg. No. _____

T. Randall M.D. _____ M.D.
Dispense as Written   Substitution Permitted

FIGURE 9-2 Sample Prescription Slip

1. The patient's name
2. The generic name of the medication
3. Both the trade and generic names if a trade name is used
4. Either the manufacturer's name or the numbers to identify the manufacturer
5. Indications of use (instructions regarding the dosage and/or strength, frequency, and route by which to administer the medication)
6. The prescription number
7. The number of refills permitted
8. Expiration date
9. Physician's name
10. Quantity in container

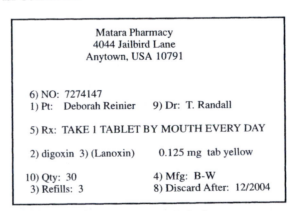

Matara Pharmacy
4044 Jailbird Lane
Anytown, USA 10791

6) NO: 7274147
1) Pt: Deborah Reinier   9) Dr: T. Randall

5) Rx: TAKE 1 TABLET BY MOUTH EVERY DAY

2) digoxin 3) (Lanoxin)   0.125 mg tab yellow

10) Qty: 30   4) Mfg: B-W
3) Refills: 3   8) Discard After: 12/2004

FIGURE 9-3 Prescription Label

OVER-THE-COUNTER MEDICATION LABELS

The information on nonprescription products differ from prescription labels in the following ways:

1. There is no patient name, prescription number, physician's name or number of refills permitted.
2. It includes a listing of active and inactive ingredients, drug interactions, and lot or batch codes.

Like a prescription, over-the-counter prescription labels include:

1. The product/medication name.
2. The name of the manufacturer or distributor.
3. Indications of use (instructions regarding the dosage and/or strength, frequency, and route by which to administer the medication).
4. The quantity in the container.
5. Precautions or warnings, if applicable.
6. Expiration date. *Never* take or administer a medication when the label indicates an expired date.

REFILLING PRESCRIPTIONS

As stated in step 4, the physician should state the number of refills that are permitted. When a patient needs a refill, ideally he or she will call the pharmacy 1 or 2 days in advance of needing the prescription refill. The

Actives per 4 tsp:
Dextromethorphan Hydrobromide 30 mg,
Pseudoephedrine Hydrochloride 60 mg
Chlorpheniramine Maleate 4 mg,
Acetaminophen 650 mg

Inactives: Alcohol 10%, Carboxymethylcellulose Sodium
Citric Acid, FD&C Blue No. 1, FD&C Red No. 40, Flavor,
High Fructose Corn syrup, Polyethylene Glycol,
Polyethylene Oxide, Propylene Glycol, Purified Water,
Sodium Citrate, Saccharin Sodium.

112853RX   Exp 9/2005

a standard cough syrup
4 fl oz (115 ml)

maximum strength cough formula

Directions: Cup inside. Under 12 yrs: Ask physician
12 years & older: 4 tsp or 20 ml.
Repeat every 6 hours, not to exceed 4 doses per day.

WARNINGS: Do not exceed recommended dosage.
DO NOT TAKE UNLESS DIRECTED BY A DOCTOR
IF YOU HAVE: . . .

Keep out of reach of children. In case of overdose . . .

FIGURE 9-4 OTC Label

patient may also personally go to the pharmacy to request the refill. There is direct communication—electronically via a computer or fax, or per telephone conversation between the pharmacy personnel and the physician's office staff—to ensure the prescription may be refilled. The specific steps may differ for individual offices; however, the procedure is fairly routine.

Clerical Steps in Refilling a Prescription

When a patient contacts a pharmacy and requests a prescription refill, pharmacy personnel contact the physician's office to obtain authorization to refill the prescription. Steps taken at the physician's office include the following.

1. *Pull Chart:* Pulling the patient's chart to determine the last date the prescription in question was filled and how many refills have been authorized.
2. *Physician Approval:* When that information is reviewed by the physician and the physician gives authorization for a refill, the pharmacy is then called.
3. *Contact Pharmacy:* The physician's office staff convey the authorization to the pharmacy staff that it is okay to refill the prescription. Depending on the medication, refills usually provide a 30- or 90-day supply. Both facilities must adhere to strict policies and procedures during this process.
4. *Documentation:* Once the physician has given authorization for the prescription to be refilled, documentation of the refill is then entered in the patient's chart.

One method of recording this information is an individualized drug flow sheet. All pertinent information is logged in one place to facilitate documentation of refills and provide one location that lists the date the medication was ordered, the medication name, dosage, frequency, refill information, the pharmacy, and the physician authorizing the prescription (see Figure 9-5).

CHAPTER REVIEW

1. Place a check mark in front of each item needed on a physician's office prescription slip.

    _____ a. patient's birth date

    _____ b. physician's office address

    _____ c. number of authorized refills

    _____ d. patient's social security number

    _____ e. physician's DEA number

    _____ f. physician's name

    _____ g. dispense as written

    _____ h. substitution permitted

Patient's Name: _____						
	Date	**Med Ordered**	**Dosage/Frequency**	**Refills**	**Pharmacy**	**M.D.**
1.						
2.						
3.						
4.						
5.						
6.						
7.						
8.						
9.						
10.						
11.						
12.						
13.						
14.						
15.						
16.						
17.						
18.						
19.						
20.						

FIGURE 9-5   Drug flow sheet

Short Answer

2. List the information documented under Signa.

_____

_____

_____

_____

3. Explain why prescription pads must be kept in a secure location.

_____

_____

_____

_____

4. How long must the hard copy of a prescription slip be retained?

_____

_____

_____

_____

Regarding information on a prescription label, indicate if the following statements are true or false by recording a T for true or an F for false.

A prescription label provides:

_____ 5. the complete address of the physician

_____ 6. the prescription number

_____ 7. the manufacturer's name or number

_____ 8. the number of refills permitted

_____ 9. the patient's birth date

_____ 10. the quantity supplied

Indicate which of the following are *not* steps in refilling prescriptions.

_____ 11. pulling the chart

_____ 12. calling the patient

_____ 13. obtaining the pharmacist's approval

_____ 14. documentation

_____ 15. contacting the pharmacy

10

Use of Drug Reference Books

COMPETENCIES

At the end of this chapter, the student should be able to:

1. Name the most widely used drug reference book in the United States.
2. Identify the various color-coded sections of the *PDR* and state their purposes.
3. Differentiate between generic and trade names in a given list of drugs.
4. Locate given drugs in specified reference books (*PDR, American Drug Index,* and *Monthly Prescribing Index*) and list adverse reactions.
5. Locate the Poison Control Center telephone number for your area.
6. Determine the controlled substance categories according to designated symbols.
7. Describe other trademark products of the *PDR*.

CHAPTER CONTENT

Physician's Desk Reference
PDR Supplements
PDR Section Breakdown
　Examining the PDR
　Additional Information in the PDR
　Steps for Using the PDR
Additional *PDR* Reference Materials

INTRODUCTION

Next to confidentiality, nothing is more important than using up-to-date reference material. There are three drug reference books that are used most often when verifying drug information.

This chapter provides the necessary instruction for determining which reference book to use to locate information, how to use the appropriate book, and also includes a variety of learning activities to give the reader experience differentiating trade names from generic names, locating adverse effects, and verifying dosages.

Maintaining a current collection of reference books is essential in the health care field. New drugs are approved, information on other drugs is revised, and medications are discontinued on a frequent basis. An up-to-date reference collection allows medical office personnel to keep abreast of these changes, provides the necessary hardware to ensure spelling accuracy, and provides the medical transcriptionist with the necessary information for accurate transcription of medications (see Figure 10-1).

PHYSICIAN'S DESK REFERENCE

The *Physician's Desk Reference* (*PDR*), which is published annually, is an excellent drug reference. Individual pharmaceutical manufacturers supply information to be included in the *PDR*; for example, trade and generic names, sources, purposes, standard dosages available, routes, side effects, and precautions. The *PDR* includes the latest information available for over 3000 products.

PDR SUPPLEMENTS

A *PDR* supplement, published bi-annually in April and August, lists important new and revised information about products listed in the *PDR*. To enable providers to remain current, these supplements are provided to those who purchase the *PDR*. Because inclusion in the *PDR* is voluntary, it is not intended as an official standard; but since it is so widely utilized, it is imperative you understand how to use it.

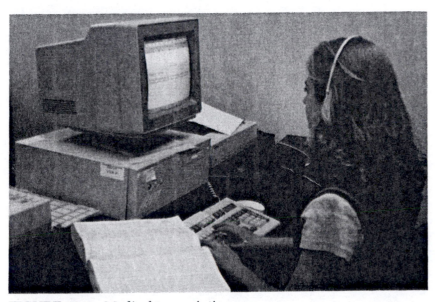

FIGURE 10-1   Medical transcription

PDR SECTION BREAKDOWN

Examining the PDR

The six sections of the *PDR* are color-coded to facilitate location of needed areas. The contents of the *PDR* are listed as follows; however, sections may vary depending on the year of the *PDR* you are using.

Section 1: Manufacturers' Index. The white pages contain an alphabetical listing of the pharmaceutical manufacturers participating in the *PDR*. These pages include prescribing information, the manufacturers' addresses, emergency contacts, and a listing of manufacturers, products, and page numbers.

Section 2: Brand and Generic Name Index. The pink section is an alphabetical listing of products by trade and generic names. When a page number is provided, you will find additional information on that product on the pages listed and a reference for the drug information section. This will probably be the most useful section to medical office personnel.

Section 3: Product Category Index. The blue pages are a quick reference section fully describing products according to the prescribing category as determined by the publisher in cooperation with each manufacturer. Examples of prescribing categories include Motion Sickness, Ophthalmic Preparations, Pain Relievers, and Laxative Drugs. Specific products are then listed under each category.

Section 4: Product Identification Section. This glossy gray section contains actual-sized, full-color reproductions of tablets, capsules, bottles, tubes, and a variety of other dosage forms and drug packages to aid in product identification. Drugs are listed alphabetically by manufacturer.

Section 5: Product Information Section. This white section is an alphabetical arrangement by manufacturer, containing over 2,500 drugs and pharmaceutical products. For most products, this section contains detailed information on drug indications and usage, dosages and routes of administration, how it is supplied, description, clinical pharmacology, warnings, contraindications, adverse reactions, precautions, generic composition, trade name, chemical name, and phonetic spelling. The generic name is listed in parentheses below the trade name.

Section 6: Diagnostic Product Information. These green pages, which list injectable materials used in radiographic diagnostic procedures and trade names of products used for lab and skin tests, are most useful to the physician.

Additional Information in the PDR

Discontinued products. This section includes a listing of discontinued products pharmaceutical companies have removed from the market during the past year.

Certified poison control centers. This is an alphabetical listing by state of the poison control centers certified by the American Association of Poison Control Centers. These facilities are open 24 hours a day, have a toll-free telephone number, are supervised by a medical director, and have registered pharmacists or nurses available to answer questions from the public.

Controlled substance categories. The symbols used to indicate the potential for abuse are provided and described. The greater the abuse potential, the more severe their prescription limitations.

Key to FDA use-in-pregnancy ratings. These ratings range from "A" to "D" and "X". These categories are based on the degree to which available information has ruled out risk to the fetus, weighed against the drug's potential benefits to the patient.

Adverse event reporting system (VAERS) forms. Health care providers and manufacturers are required by law to complete a VAERS form on each patient who experiences a reaction to a vaccine listed in the Injury Table (see Figure 10-2). Health care providers and manufacturers who observe suspect reactions to any drug or biologics administered are required to fill out a Reporting Adverse Reactions Form (see Figure 10-3.) The completed form is mailed to the FDA in Rockville, Maryland.

Steps for Using the PDR

When transcribing dictation, the physician will occasionally spell the drug name. This does not mean, however, the spelling is accurate. It is imperative the medical secretary or medical transcriptionist double-check to verify the spelling accuracy. There are numerous look-alike sound-alike drugs. The importance of accuracy in drug transcription cannot be overstressed.

It significantly increases the chances of transcribing the correct medication if the transcriptionist has the patient's chart in his or her position. This is not always feasible, however. Drug reference books are the most valuable resources for verifying accurate spelling, double-checking a dictator's mumbled dosage or frequency, determining if the dictator truly meant what he or she said, and locating other essential drug information.

For the medical secretary and medical transcriptionist, the pink section (the Brand and Generic Name Index), will be the most useful. Again, this section is an alphabetical listing of products. If after review of the pink section you are not completely convinced that the medication you have transcribed is correct, follow through to the page number provided in the pink section. Read the information provided to help determine the correct medication. Questions to ask yourself to verify drug accuracy are:

1. Would that medication be prescribed for the conditions or diagnoses dictated?
2. If a dosage was dictated, is it consistent with the dosages provided?
3. If the frequency was dictated, is it consistent with the frequencies provided?

VACCINE ADVERSE EVENT REPORTING SYSTEM
24 Hour Toll-free information line 1-800-822-7967
P.O. Box 1100, Rockville, MD 20849-1100
PATIENT IDENTITY KEPT CONFIDENTIAL

VAERS

For CDC/FDA Use Only

VAERS Number _____

Date Received _____

Patient Name:	*Vaccine administered by (Name):*	*Form completed by (Name):*
Last First M.I.	Responsible Physician _____	Relation ☐ Vaccine Provider ☐ Patient Parent to Patient ☐ Manufacturer ☐ Other
Address	Facility Name/Address	Address (if different from patient or provider)
City State Zip	City State Zip	City State Zip
Telephone no. (___) _____	Telephone no. (___) _____	Telephone no. (___) _____

1. State	2. County where administered	3. Date of birth ___/___/___ mm dd yy	4. Patient age	5. Sex ☐M ☐F	6. Date form completed ___/___/___ mm dd yy

7. Describe adverse events(s) (symptoms, signs, time course) and treatment, if any

8. Check all appropriate:
☐ Patient died   (date ___/___/___)
☐ Life threatening illness   mm dd yy
☐ Required emergency room/doctor visit
☐ Required hospitalization (_____days)
☐ Resulted in prolongation of hospitalization
☐ Resulted in permanent disability
☐ None of the above

9. Patient recovered ☐YES ☐NO ☐UNKNOWN	10. Date of vaccination ___/___/___ mm dd yy Time _____ AM PM	11. Adverse event onset ___/___/___ mm dd yy Time _____ AM PM

12. Relevant diagnostic tests/laboratory data

13. Enter all vaccines given on date listed in no. 10

	Vaccine (type)	Manufacturer	Lot number	Route/Site	No. Previous Doses
a.					
b.					
c.					
d.					

14. Any other vaccinations within 4 weeks prior to the date listed in no. 10

	Vaccine (type)	Manufacturer	Lot number	Route/Site	No. Previous doses	Date given
a.						
b.						

15. Vaccinated at: ☐ Private doctor's office/hospital ☐ Military clinic/hospital ☐ Public health clinic/hospital ☐ Other/unknown	16. Vaccine purchased with: ☐ Private funds ☐ Military funds ☐ Public funds ☐ Other/unknown	17. Other medications

18. Illness at time of vaccination (specify)	19. Pre-existing physician-diagnosed allergies, birth defects, medial conditions (specify)

20. Have you reported this adverse event previously?	☐ No ☐ To doctor	☐ To health department ☐ To manufacturer	**Only for children 5 and under**

22. Birth weight _____ lb. _____ oz.	23. No. of brothers and sisters

21. Adverse event following prior vaccination (check all applicable, specify)

	Adverse Event	Onset Age	Type Vaccine	Dose no. in series
☐ In patient				
☐ In brother or sister				

Only for reports submitted by manufacturer/immunization project

24. Mfr./imm. proj. report no.	25. Date received by mfr./imm. proj.
26. 15 day report? ☐ Yes ☐ No	27. Report type ☐ Initial ☐ Follow-Up

Health care providers and manufacturers are required by law (42 USC 300aa-25) to report reactions to vaccines listed in the Table of Reportable Events Following Immunization. Reports for reactions to other vaccines are voluntary except when required as a condition of immunization grant awards.

Form VAERS-1(FDA)

FIGURE 10-2 Form VAERS-1

Form Approved: OMB No. 0910-0291 Expires: 4/30/96
See OMB statement on reverse

MEDWATCH

THE FDA MEDICAL PRODUCTS REPORTING PROGRAM

For **VOLUNTARY** reporting
by health professionals of adverse
events and product problems

Page _____ of _____

FDA Use only

Triage unit
sequence #

A. Patient information

1. Patient identifier	2. Age at time of event: or Date of birth	3. Sex	4. Weight
In confidence		☐ Male ☐ Female	_____ lbs or _____ kgs

B. Adverse event or product problem

☐ Adverse event   and/or   ☐ Product problem (e.g., defects/malfunctions)

1. Outcomes attributed to adverse event (check all that apply)

☐ death _____ (mo/day/yr)
☐ life-threatening
☐ hospitalization – initial or prolonged

☐ disability
☐ congenital anomaly
☐ required intervention to prevent permanent impairment/damage
☐ other: _____

2. Date of event (mo/day/yr)	3. Date of this report (mo/day/yr)

Describe event or problem

Relevant tests/laboratory data, including dates

Other relevant history, including preexisting medical conditions (e.g., allergies, race, pregnancy, smoking and alcohol use, hepatic/renal dysfunction, etc.)

C. Suspect medication(s)

1. Name (give labeled strength & mfr/labeler, if known)

#1

#2

2. Dose, frequency & route used	3. Therapy dates (if unknown, give duration) from/to (or best estimate)
#1	#1
#2	#2

4. Diagnosis for use (indication)	5. Event abated after use stopped or dose reduced
#1	#1 ☐ yes ☐ no ☐ doesn't apply
#2	#2 ☐ yes ☐ no ☐ doesn't apply

6. Lot # (if known)	6. Exp. date (if known)	7. Event reappeared after reintroduction
#1	#1	#1 ☐ yes ☐ no ☐ doesn't apply
#2	#2	#2 ☐ yes ☐ no ☐ doesn't apply

9. NDC # (for product problems only)

10. Concomitant medical products and terapy dates (exclude treatment of event)

D. Suspect medical device

1. Brand name

2. Type of device

3. Manufacturer name & address	4. Operator of device
	☐ Health professional ☐ lay user/patient ☐ Other _____

6. model # _____ catalog # _____ serial # _____ lot # _____ other #	5. Expiration date (mo/day/year)
	7. If implanted, give date (mo/day/year)
	8. If explanted, give date (mo/day/year)

9. Device available for evaluation? (Do not send to FDA)

☐ yes   ☐ no   ☐ returned to manufacturer on _____ (mo/day/year)

10. Concomitant medical products and therapy dates (exclude treatment of event)

E. Reporter (see confidentiality section on back)

1. Name & address	phone #

2. Health professional? ☐ yes ☐ no	3. Occupation	4. Also reported to ☐ manufacturer ☐ user facility ☐ distributor
5. If you do NOT want your identity disclosed to the manufacturer, place an "X" in this box. ☐		

FDA

Mail to: MEDWATCH
5600 Fishers Lane
Rockville, MD 20852-9787

or **FAX to:**
1-800-FDA-0178

FDA Form 3500

Submission of a report does not constitute an admission that medical personnel or the product caused or contributed to the event.

FIGURE 10-3 FDA Form 3500 for Voluntary Reporting of Adverse Events

Are all answers to these questions yes? If so, then you can be comfortable the drug is accurate. If you have answered no to any of these questions, your work is not finished. If you have exhausted the drug reference books available and you are still not comfortable that the drug transcribed is accurate, the progress note or report you are transcribing must be flagged and brought to the attention of the dictator for clarification. *Never guess* when transcribing a medication. Remember, inclusion of products in the *PDR* is strictly voluntary. It only lists those drugs the pharmaceutical companies pay to have listed; therefore, not every medication is included.

ADDITIONAL PDR REFERENCE MATERIALS

In addition to the *PDR*, there are *PDR for Non-Prescription Drugs, PDR for Ophthalmology*, electronic devices such as Pocket PDR, and PDR Library on CD-ROM for personal computers.

There are also many additional sources of drug information available, such as the *American Drug Index*, published annually, and the *Monthly Prescribing Reference*, which is published monthly. It is vital you become aware of what is readily accessible, always maintain the most up-to-date reference books, and use them.

CHAPTER REVIEW

Short Answer

1. How often is the *PDR* published? _____

    _____

    _____

    _____

    _____

2. How often is the *PDR* supplement published?_____

    _____

    _____

    _____

    _____

3. What section of the *PDR* will the medical secretary find most useful?_____

    _____

    _____

    _____

    _____

4. Draw a line from the section descriptions to the correct color coding.

pink section   Manufacturers' Index

blue section   Brand and Generic Name Index

green section   Discontinued Products

white section (emergency   Product Identification Section
contacts)
                                                Product Information Section
white section (over 2500 drugs
and pharmaceutical products)   Diagnostic Product Information

gray glossy section   Product Category Index

5. Locate the following drugs and indicate adverse effects.

a. Claritin _____

b. Paxil _____

c. Lanoxin _____

d. Coumadin _____

e. Vasotec _____

f. Cipro _____

g. Hytrin _____

h. Pepcid _____

i. Cefzil _____

j. Dilantin _____

6. Locate the following drugs and indicate if they are trade or generic names (all are intentionally listed in lowercase).

_____ a. phenytoin

_____ b. relafen

_____ c. accupril

_____ d. ortho-novum 7/7/7

_____ e. atenolol

_____ f. cardizem cd

_____ g. premarin

_____ h. tenormin

_____ i. duricef

_____ j. zestril

11

Drug Classifications, Actions, and Examples

COMPETENCIES

At the end of this chapter, the student should be able to:

1. Determine the drug classification of specified drugs using reference books.
2. Explain the action on the body when a drug of a specific classification is administered.
3. Name the two major divisions of pain relievers.
4. Explain the differences among specific over-the-counter (OTC) pain relievers.
5. Give brand name examples of the five types of OTC pain relievers.
6. Define NSAIDs.
7. Explain the possible side effects of OTC drugs.

CHAPTER CONTENT

Drug Classifications
Analgesics
Nonnarcotic Painkillers
Narcotic Painkillers

INTRODUCTION

To properly verify that the medication in question is correct, it is essential to know drug classifications and the drug's action on the body. This chapter provides an alphabetical listing of drug classifications, the corresponding body response from taking a medication in that particular class, and examples of medications in each class. Another very important part of this chapter is a listing of the most commonly prescribed medications and the drug classifications in which they fall.

DRUG CLASSIFICATIONS

Now that you have completed chapters 1 through 10, you are ready to learn the various drug classifications and the effects such drugs have on the body. Table 1 provides a listing of drug classifications followed by the drug action. An alphabetical listing of commonly used drugs is provided in Table 2. Please note this is not an inclusive listing of medications, but a list of drugs used on a regular basis.

In some instances, you may need to locate a medication by utilizing the drug classification. In other circumstances you may need to use an alphabetical listing to locate the specific name of a medication. Table 11-2, a list indexed by drug name, also includes the drug classification.

ANALGESICS

One last area to be covered is one that can be very confusing to the average person—analgesics (painkillers that give temporary relief without causing loss of consciousness).

Pain is universal and unique. Approximately half of all Americans seek treatment for pain each year. Although pain can be beneficial by alerting you to injury when you break a bone, it can also be relentlessly overwhelming. With the advancements in medicine, pain need no longer be a companion of a disease. Pain often originates in nerve receptors called nociceptors. Upon receiving stimuli such as pressure, temperature change, inflammation, infection, disease, or injury, the receptors instantly notify the central nervous system of these changes, allowing us to feel the pain emotionally and psychologically. Some individuals can tolerate pain to a higher degree. Regardless of what your pain threshold is, ideally we would rather *not* experience pain. Once it is determined why there is pain, it can often be controlled with use of medications. A variety of drug delivery systems help provide effective pain relief. There are drug-free methods such as electrical stimulation, acupuncture, cryotherapy, thermotherapy, and whirlpool baths. An easier, less expensive method of pain control, however, is use of over-the-counter pain relievers.

There are two major divisions of painkillers: nonnarcotics and narcotics.

Nonnarcotic Painkillers

Nonnarcotic (over-the-counter, or **OTC**) painkillers are the most widely used of all medications. Despite the fact they are sold over the counter, OTC pain relievers are serious medicines. It is imperative you always read and follow the labeled directions, take only the recommended dosage, be aware of any contraindications, and never mix medications with alcohol.

OTC pain relievers are broken down into five categories, based on the active ingredient. Refer to Table 11-3 for a thumbnail sketch of OTC pain relievers.

TABLE 11-1

Drug Classification	Action on Body	Examples of Drugs
alpha blocker	Relaxes blood vessels	Minipress, prazosin
amphetamine	Acts as stimulant on central nervous system; has temporary effect of increasing energy and mental alertness; sometimes used to depress the appetite	Amphetamine sulfate, Dexedrine, Desoxyn, Ritalin, Preluden
analgesic	Relieves pain without loss of consciousness	acetaminophen (Tylenol), aspirin, ibuprofen (Advil, Motrin), Talwin, Naproxen, Darvon-N, Darvon
anesthetic	Produces generalized or local loss of feeling by interfering with conduction of nerve impulses	Locals: lidocaine HCl (Xylocaine) procaine HCl (Novocain), Nupercaine, Marcaine, Nesacaine Generals: Pentothal sodium, halothane (Fluothane), nitrous oxide, Ketalar, Brevital, Amidate, cyclopropane
antacid	Neutralizes stomach acidity	Amphojel, Gelusil, Mylanta, MOM, Tums, Rolaids, Riopan, Gaviscon, Maalox, Tagamet, Pepcid, Zantac
antianaphylactic	Prevents anaphylaxis; desensitization	Ana-Kit, Alferon N, Cyto-Gam, Gammar
antianginal agent	Relieves heart and chest pain associated with angina	Sorbitrate, nitroglycerin, Lopressor, Nitrogard, Nitrostat, Indural, Isoptin, Isordil, Peritrate, Cardizem, Corgard, diltiazem, Tenormin, verapamil
antianxiety agents	Relieves anxiety and muscle tension; minor tranquilizers	diazepam, Valium, Librium, Xanax, Ativan, Tranxene
antiarrhythmic	Acts to control or prevent cardiac arrhythmias	lidocaine HCl (Xylocaine) propranolol HCl (Inderal)
antiarthritic	Acts against arthritic problems	lidocaine HCl (Xylocaine HCl), propranolol (Inderal), Extentabs, Procan SR
antibiotic	Fights infection, inhibits growth, or causes death of microorganisms	penicillin (Pentids, Pen-Vee K, Duracillin) cephalosporins (Keflin, Rocephin), ampicillin (Polycillin, Amacill), amoxicillin (Amoxil)

TABLE 11-1 (continued)

Drug Classification	Action on Body	Examples of Drugs
anticholinergic	Opposes the action of acetylcholine; blocks parasympathetic nerve impulses	scopolamine, Artane, Atropisol, Propine, Cyclogyl
anticoagulant	Prevents or delays blood clotting	heparin, dicumarol, warfarin sodium (Coumadin)
anticonvulsant	Relieves, prevents, or treats seizures	Tegretol, Dilantin, Zarontin, Diamox, Valium, Mysoline
antidepressant	Prevents or relieves depression; often called mood elevator	Prozac, Asendin, Marplan, Nardil, Elavil, Tofranil
antidiabetic agents	Prevents or relieves diabetes	Orinase, Tolinase, insulin
antidiarrheal	Prevents or counteracts diarrhea	Lomotil, Pepto-Bismol, Kaopectate, Imodium
antidote	Neutralizes or counteracts poison	naloxone (Narcan)
antidiuretic	Lessens or decreases urine secretion	DDAVP nasal spray, DDAVP rhinal tube, DDAVP tablets
antiemetic	Prevents or counteracts nausea and vomiting; used to treat vertigo and motion sickness	Tigan, Dramamine, Phenergan, Reglan, Marinol, Thorazine, Benadryl, Antivert, Transderm-scop
antifungal	Treats fungal infections	Diflucan, Monistat 3, Mycelex vaginal tabs, Vagistat-1
antihistamine	Prevents or diminishes the effects of histamine; given to relieve symptoms of seasonal allergies such as hay fever, and also to relieve symptoms of the common cold such as stuffy nose and itchy eyes	Dimetane, Benadryl, Seldane, Optimine, Dimetane, Chlor-Trimeton, Tavist
antihypertensive (hypotensive)	Controls or lowers high blood pressure	Lasix, Aldactone, Aldomet, Catapres, Lopressor, Apresoline, Capoten, Aldoril, Tenex, Isoptin SR, Minipres, atenolol (Tenormin)
anti-inflammatory agent (corticosteroid)	Reduces or relieves inflammation	naproxen (Naprosyn), aspirin, ibuprofen (Advil, Motrin); see corticosteroids for more

TABLE 11-1 (continued)

Drug Classification	Action on Body	Examples of Drugs
antilipemic	Lowers high levels of fatty substances in blood	Nicolar, Nicobid, Lopid, Colestid, Lipitor, Zocor, Pravachol, Questran, Lorelco
antimanic	Treats manic-depressive disorders and bipolar disorders	Lithium
antimetabolites	Interferes with the metabolic process, preventing all reproduction	Tabloid, 5-FU, Cytosar
antineoplastic	Inhibits growth and spread of malignant cells	cisplatin (Platinol), Thioplex, busulfan (Myleran), cyclophosphamide (Cytoxan)
antiparkinsonian	Palliative relief of bradykinesia, rigidity, tremors, and problems with equilibrium and posture	Symmetrel, Cogentin, Sinemet, Dopar, Artane
antipsychotic	Treat schizophrenia, paranoia, and other psychotic disorders	Thorazine, Mellaril, Compazine, Trilafon, haloperidol (Haldol), Navane
antipruritic	Prevents or relieves itching; may be a drug, ointment, or solution	Atarax, Tavist
antipyretic	Lowers body temperature; reduces fever	aspirin (Bayer), acetaminophen (Tylenol), ibuprofen (Advil, Motrin, Nuprin), naproxen (Naprosyn)
antirheumatics	Treats rheumatoid arthritis by reducing pain, swelling, and stiffness; a gold compound	Ridaura
antispasmodic	Stops spasm of voluntary or involuntary muscles (like the peristaltic activity) of the GI tract	Bentyl, Levsin, Daricon, Pathilon
antitussive	Prevents or relieves cough	codeine, codeine sulfate, Dicodid, Codone, codeine phosphate, hydrobromide, Benylin, Tessalon
antiviral	Treats viral infections	Videx, ganciclovir sodium, zidovudine (AZT), Viroptic, Zovirax
astringent	Constricts tissue or mucous membranes and decreases or arrests minor hemorrhage and reduces perspiration and other secretions	Salts of aluminum, zinc, and other heavy metals, tannic acid in alcohol, witch hazel

TABLE 11-1   (continued)

Drug Classification	Action on Body	Examples of Drugs
ataractic	See *tranquilizers*	
barbiturates	Relieves anxiety, treats insomnia, and controls epilepsy; used medically as sedatives	pentobarbital (Nembutal), secobarbital (Seconal), phenobarbital (Luminal), Amytal, Alurate
beta blocker	Slows heart; decreases force of heartbeat	acebutolol (Secral), Cartrol, Levatol, Inderal, Lopressor, Tenormin, Corgard
bronchodilator	Relaxes and dilates the bronchi to increase air flow	Isuprel, Proventil, Ventolin, Adrenalin, Bricanyl, theophylline (Theo-24), Choledyl
calcium channel blocker	Relaxes blood vessels (helpful for angina)	Procardia, verapamil (Calan), diltiazem HCl (Cardizem)
cardiac glycosides	Treats heart failures; digitalis compounds	digitoxin (Digitoline), digoxin (Lanoxin)
cathartics	Relieves constipation and promotes defecation; strong laxative	Dulcolax, Colace, MOM, Ex-Lax, Metamucil
contraceptive	Prevents or diminishes likelihood of conception	Enovid-E 21, Ortho-Novum, Demulen 1/50-21, Ovulen-28
corticosteroid	Used to decrease inflammation and treat allergic rhinitis; topical or oral drug. See *anti-inflammatory agent*	prednisone, Urtcort, Valisone, Topicort, Decaderm, Decadron phosphate, Cortef, Haldron. Inhalational corticosteroids: Decadron, Aerobid, Azmacort, Beclovent
decongestant	Treats nasal congestion; constricts dilated arterioles reducing nasal blood flow, improving drainage	Afrin, Neo-Synephrine, Sudafed, Sinutab sinus spray
diuretic	Decreases kidney reabsorption, causing increased amounts of salt and water excreted in urine; reduces fluid retention; treats edema and hypertension	Diamox, Diuril, Lasix, Enduron, Aldactone, Osmitrol
emetic	Stimulates vomiting; usually for those having overdosed or ingested poison	Ipecac syrup

TABLE 11-1 (continued)

Drug Classification	Action on Body	Examples of Drugs
estrogen supplement	Treats amenorrhea and dysfunctional bleeding; palliative treatment for breast cancer and prostate cancer; given for symptoms accompanying menopause	Premarin, Estrace, Menest, Estinyl, Estrovis
expectorant	Liquefies mucus in bronchi and aids in the expectoration of sputum, mucus, and phlegm; relieves and suppresses cough	Robitussin, terpin hydrate elixir, Mucomyst
fertility drugs	Increases the chances of impregnation	clomiphene (Clomid)
hemostatic	Controls or arrests flow of blood by helping coagulation	Humafac, Amicar, vitamin K
hormone	Endocrine system produces hormones and secretes them directly into bloodstream; commercial preps are available; act in same manner as naturally occurring hormones	Estrogen, Premarin, androgens, progestins (Megace), adrenal corticosteroids (prednisone)
hypnotic	Produces sleep or hypnosis; includes analgesics, anesthetics, and intoxicants	secobarbital (Seconal), Placidyl
hypoglycemic	Lowers blood glucose level	Diabinese, DiaBeta, Tolinase, Orinase, insulin
immunosuppressive	Suppresses body's natural immune response to antigen; interferes with the body systems that resist infection and foreign materials	Imuran, Rhogam
insulin preparations	Essential for the proper metabolism of blood sugar (glucose) and for maintenance of the proper blood sugar level; used to treat diabetes	regular, semilente, NPH, Lente, Humulin R
laxative	Loosens and promotes movement of bowels; relieves constipation	See *cathartics*
miotic	Contracts pupil of eye	Pilocar ophthalmic solution, pilocarpine

TABLE 11-1   (continued)

Drug Classification	Action on Body	Examples of Drugs
muscle relaxant	Produces relaxation of skeletal muscles; relieves spasms	Paraflex, Flexeril, Valium, Robaxin, Norflex, Skelaxin, Atropisol, Cyclogyl, Glaucon, Naphcon, Neo-Synephrine
mydriatic	Dilates pupil of eye	atropine, ephedrine
narcotic	Produces sound sleep, stupor, and relief of pain; also referred to as opiate	morphine, codeine, Demerol, Dilaudid
nonsteroidal anti-inflammatory drugs (NSAIDs)	Drugs used to treat inflammation and arthritis	See *anti-inflammatory agent*
placebo	Exerts no pharmacologic action, no therapeutic effect, and produces no side effects; commonly sugar pills or injections of sterile normal saline solution. Although it is physiologically impossible for a placebo to exert any pharmacologic effect, patients often report a decrease of symptoms when given a placebo. This demonstrates that the power of suggestion can produce changes within the body which closely mimic the pharmacologic action of a drug.	Drug name is often mutually agreed upon by physician and pharmacist
Progestins	Prevents uterine bleeding; treats amenorrhea, infertility, and threatened or habitual miscarriage	Provera, Norlutin, Gesterol
prophylaxis	Prevents the development of a disease or other condition such as birth control pills, hormones, vaccines, or vitamins	birth control pill: Ortho Novum *7/7/7* vaccine: HIB, MMR vitamin: Tri-Vi-Flor
psychedelic	Produces feelings of relaxation, freedom from anxiety, highly creative thought patterns and perceptual changes; causes hallucinations; alters mental functions. Highly controversial, potentially very dangerous, and used only under controlled supervision for experimental purposes.	LSD, mescaline

TABLE 11-1 (continued)

Drug Classification	Action on Body	Examples of Drugs
sedative	Quiets and relaxes patient; relieves anxiety without inducing sleep	Nonbarbituate sedative-hypnotics: Placidyl, Dalmane, Doriden, Restoril, Halcion. For barbituate sedative-hypnotics see *barbituates*.
stimulant	Increases the activity of the CNS	caffeine, Benzedrine, Metrazol, Dopram, Ritalin
styptic	Arrests bleeding by means of astringent (binding or coagulation) quality	alum (is OTC)
sulfonamide (sulfa preparation)	Fights a variety of bacterial infections	Gantrisin, Gantanol, Bactrim, Septra
tranquilizers (also called ataractics)	Relieves anxiety and tension; calms or quiets patient without interfering with normal mental activity or affecting the stimulation that antidepressants produce	Thorazine, Mellaril, Haldol
vaccine	Produces immunity and prevents infectious diseases	diphtheria, polio, tetanus (DPT), HIB, MMR, influenza virus, hepatitis B
vasoconstrictor	Constricts blood vessels to increase force of heartbeat; relieves nasal congestion, raises BP, and stops superficial hemorrhages	Adrenalin, Levophed, Aramine
vasopressor	Produces contraction of arteries and capillaries; elevates blood pressure	Intropin, Aramine, Neo-Synephrine 1% injections, norepinephrine (Levophed)
vasodilator	Relaxes and dilates blood vessels, which increases blood flow and reduces blood pressure	Isordil, Serpasil, nitroglycerin, sorbitrate
vitamins	Necessary for the body to grow and maintain health; organic substances found in foods. Commercial preps of most vitamins are available. They are required for normal growth and development.	Fat-soluble: vitamin A, D, E, K Water-soluble: vitamin B1, B2, B6, B12, C

TABLE 11-2   FREQUENTLY USED DRUGS AND DRUG CLASSIFICATIONS

DRUG	DRUG CLASSIFICATION
5-FU (fluorouracil)	antimetabolite
acebutolol	beta blocker
acetaminophen	analgesic
Actifed	antihistamine; decongestant
Adrenalin	bronchodilator; antianaphylactic; vasoconstrictor; adrenergic
Advil	analgesic
alcohol	antiseptic (skin)
Aldactazide	antihypertensive
Aldactone	diuretic; antihypertensive
Alkeran	antineoplastic
allopurinol	gout treatment, arthritis; miscellaneous prep, uninary system
alprozolam	tranquilizer
aminophylline	bronchodilator
amoxicillin	antibiotic
ampicillin	antibiotic
Antivert	antiemetic
Apresoline	vasodilator; antihypertensive
aspirin	analgesic
Atarax	antianxiety; antihistamine; antipruritic
Azulfidine	antibiotic
Bactrim	antibiotic; anti-infective (urinary); sulfa prep
belladonna	antispasmodic
Benadryl	antihistamine; sedative
Benylin	expectorant (cough medication)
caffeine	stimulant
Cardizem	antianginal; calcium channel blocker
Cardura	alpha blocker; hypertension
castor oil	cathartic; laxative
Catapres	antihypertensive
cefazolin	antibiotic
cefotaxime	antibiotic
cephalexin	antibiotic
cephalosporin	antibiotic
Chlor-trimeton	antihistamine
chloral hydrate	hypnotic
chlordiazepoxide	tranquilizer
cimetidine	antacid, ulcer and reflux treatment
Claritin	antihistamine
Clomid	gonadotropic; fertility drug
codeine	antidiarrheal; analgesic; narcotic; expectorant
Colace	laxative

TABLE 11-2 (continued)

DRUG	DRUG CLASSIFICATION
Compazine	antianxiety; tranquilizer; antiemetic; GI
Corgard	antianginal; beta blocker
cortisone	anti-inflammatory; hormone
Coumadin	anticoagulant
Cytoxan	antineoplastic
Dalmane	sedative
Darvocet-N	analgesic
Darvon	analgesic
Decadron	nasal prep; antiallergic; otic
Demerol	narcotic
Dexedrin	amphetamine; stimulant
Diabeta	hypoglycemic
Diabinese	antidiabetic; hypoglycemic
Dialose	cathartic; laxative
Diamox	diuretic
digitalis	antiarrhythmic; cardiogenic
digitoxin	antiarrhythmic; cardiogenic
digoxin	antiarrhythmic; cardiogenic
Dilantin	anticonvulsant
diltiazem	antianginal; calcium channel blocker
Dimetane	antihistamine (cough medication)
Diuril	diuretic
Donnatal	antispasmodic; antacid; ulcer and reflux treatment
Doxidan	laxative
Dramamine	antiemetic
Dulcolax	cathartic; laxative
Dyazide	diuretic; antihypertensive
Elavil	antidepressant
Empirin with codeine	analgesic
Enduron	antihypertensive; diuretic
Enovid	gonadotropic; contraceptive
ephedrine sulfate	vasoconstrictor
epinephrine	adrenergic
epinephrine	antianaphylactic; adrenergic; vasoconstrictor
Equanil	antianxiety; tranquilizer
Erythrocin	antibiotic
erythromycin	antibiotic
Esidrix	antihypertensive; diuretic
estrogen	hormone
Euthroid	hormone
Flagyl	antibiotic; antibacterial; amebicide
Fleet enema	laxative

TABLE 11-2 (continued)

DRUG	DRUG CLASSIFICATION
Furadantin	anti-infective (urinary)
Gantrisin	sulfa prep
Garamycin	anti-infective; antifungal; antibiotic; ophthalmic
Gaviscon	antacid; GI
Gelucil	antacid
gentamicin	antibiotic
Halcion	sedative
Haldol	antipsychotic (major tranquilizer)
Haley's MO	laxative
Halotestin	hormone
heparin	anticoagulant
hydralazine	vasodilator
hydrochlorothiazide (HCTZ)	diuretic
ibuprofen	analgesic
Imodium	antidiarrheal; GI
Imuran	immunosuppressant
Inderal	antianginal; antihypertensive
Indocin	anti-inflammatory; antiarthritic
insulin	hormone; antidiabetic; hypoglycemia
Ipecac syrup	emetic; antidote
Ismelin	antihypertensive
Isoptin	antianginal; calcium channel blocker
Isordil	antianginal agent
Isuprel	antiasthmatic; bronchodilator
K-Lor	potassium supplement
K-Lyte	potassium supplement
Kaopectate	antidiarrheal
KCl	potassium supplement
Keflex	antibiotic
Kenocort	anti-inflammatory
Kenalog	anti-inflammatory
Kondremul	laxative
Lanoxin	cardiogenic
Lasix	diuretic; antihypertensive
Lente insulin	antidiabetic
Leukeran	antineoplastic
Librax	antispasmodic
Librium	antianxiety (minor tranquilizer)
lithium	tranquilizer
Lomotil	antidiarrheal
Lopressor	antianginal; beta blocker; antihypertensive
LSD	psychedelic

TABLE 11-2   (continued)

DRUG	DRUG CLASSIFICATION
Maalox	antacid
meclizine	antiemetic
Mefoxin	antibiotic
Megace	chemotherapy
Mellaril	antipsychotic (major tranquilizer)
mescaline	psychedelic
Metamucil	laxative
methotrexate	antineoplastic
Midamor	diuretic; antihypertensive
Milk of Magnesia	cathartic; laxative
mineral oil	cathartic; laxative
Minipress	antihypertensive; alpha blocker
MOPP	chemotherapy
morphine	narcotic; analgesic
Mycostatin	anti-infective/antifungal
Mylanta	antacid
NegGram	anti-infective (urinary)
Nembutal	sedative
Neosporin	anti-infective/antifungal; ophthalmic
Neo-Synephrine	nasal prep; decongestant
Nitrogard	antianginal
nitroglycerin	antianginal; vasodilator (cardiovascular)
Nitrostat	antianginal
NuLYTELY	laxative
Nuprin	antiarthritic; anti-inflammatory
Orinase	antidiabetic; hypoglycemic
Ornade Spansule	decongestant
Ortho-Novum	contraceptive
Orudis	antiarthritic; analgesic
paregoric	antidiarrheal
Pen Vee K	antibiotic
penicillin V	antibiotic
Percodan	analgesic
Peri-Colace	laxative
Peritrate	antianginal; vasodilator
Phenergan	antihistamine; antiemetic
phenobarbital	sedative; anticonvulsant
Pilocar ophthalmic solution	miotic
pilocarpine	miotic
pontocaine hydrochloride	anesthetic
prazosin	alpha blocker; antihypertensive
prednisone	corticosteroid; such a widely used medication, falls into numerous general categories

TABLE 11-2   (continued)

DRUG	DRUG CLASSIFICATION
Premarin	estrogen supplement; gonadotropic
Procan	antiarrhythmic
Procardia	antianginal; calcium channel blocker
progesterone	hormone
Pronestyl	cardiogenic
Prozac	antidepressant
quinidine	antiarrhythmic
reserpine	antihypertensive
Restoril	sedative
Ridaura	antiarthritic
Riopan	antacid
Ritalin	attention deficit disorder
Robitussin	expectorant (cough medication)
Salk polio vaccine	vaccine
secobarbital	sedative
Seconal	sedative
Selsun	antiseborrheic
Senokot	laxative
Septra	antibiotic
Serpasil	antihypertensive; vasodilator
Slow-K	potassium supplement
sodium bicarbonate	antacid
sodium warfarin	anticoagulant
Soma compound	muscle relaxant
Sorbitrate	vasodilator; antianginal
streptomycin	antibiotic
stypic pencil	styptic
Sudafed	decongestant
Tagamet	GI (ulcers)
temoxifen	antineoplastic
Tavist	antipruritic
Tenormin	beta blocker; antianginal
testosterone	hormone
tetanus shot	vaccine
Thorazine	antipsychotic (major tranquilizer)
Tigan	antiemetic
Tofranil	antidepressant
Tolinase	antidiabetic; hypoglycemic
triazolam	hypnotic; sedative
Tylenol	analgesic; antipyretic
typhoid vaccine	vaccine
V-cillin K	antibiotic
Valium	antianxiety (minor tranquilizer); muscle relaxant

TABLE 11-2 (continued)

DRUG	DRUG CLASSIFICATION
vasopressin	antidiuretic
verapamil	antianginal; calcium channel blocker; antihypertensive
vitamin B, C	water soluble vitamins
vitamin A, D, E, K	fat soluble vitamins
vitamin K	hemostatic
warfarin	anticoagulant
Xanax	antianxiety; tranquilizer
xylocaine hydrochloride	anesthetic
Zantac	antacid, ulcer and reflux treatment
zofran	antiemetic; usually for chemotherapy patients
Zostrix	topical analgesic

These painkillers not only control pain, but depending on the analgesic, can also lower fever and counter inflammation. While all four analgesics will relieve minor pain (headaches, toothaches, muscle aches, arthritis, and menstrual cramps), they are also antipyretics, or fever reducers. Pain relievers are most effective when you match the drug with your symptoms. One subtle difference among the categories is in reducing inflammation.

NSAIDs. Aspirin, ibuprofen, and naproxen sodium are nonsteroidal anti-inflammatory drugs (**NSAIDs**). They may be used as anti-inflammatory drugs on a long-term basis, unlike steroids, which can cause serious side effects.

Using OTC pain relievers is not as simple as it sounds. You must match the pill to the pain. When you do not need an anti-inflammatory, acetaminophen is a safe pain reliever, but should be used with caution by persons with liver or kidney disorders. *Do not* combine aspirin and acetaminophen, as it is damaging to the kidneys. Special risks are listed under Drug Effects in chapter 4. A secondary effect of aspirin is that when taken in low doses, it may help prevent a heart attack or stroke by preventing clot formation. Table 11-3 provides a partial listing of NSAIDs available in prescription and/or OTC form. Because people respond differently to each medication, it may be necessary to try several before finding the one that works best for you. NSAIDs may cause GI bleeding and stomach upset; however, to minimize these side effects, they are to be taken with food or milk.

There is a significant difference in price for OTC pain relievers. Typically, you can buy generic regular strength aspirin for approximately 2 cents per pill. The same aspirin with an antacid costs about 13 cents each, and it increases to 15 cents for an effervescing antacid. Whereas the aspirin is 2 cents, the acetaminophen tab is approximately 5 cents, ibuprofen 6 to 7 cents, and naproxen sodium slightly more than ibuprofen.

TABLE 11-3 OVER-THE-COUNTER PAIN RELIEVERS

	aspirin	acetaminophen	ibuprofen	naproxen sodium	ketoprofen
Examples of name brands:	Anacin Ascriptin Bayer Bufferin	aspirin-free Excedrin aspirin-free Anacin Tylenol	Advil Motrin Motrin IB Nuprin	Aleve Anaprox Naprosyn	Actron Orudis Orudis KT Oruvail
Anti-inflammatory: (Nonsteroidal anti-inflammatory drugs/NSAIDs)	Yes	No	Yes	Yes	Yes
Antipyrexia:	Yes	Yes	Yes	Yes	Yes
Possible side effects:	GI bleed, stomach upset, or ulceration	None when taken as directed, less likely to cause stomach upset	GI bleed, stomach upset, ulceration, or pain	GI bleed, stomach upset, bloating, or dizziness	GI upset
	Not recommended for those under age 16	Preferred choice for those under age 16			Not recommended for children under 16 years of age

SPECIAL NOTES: If you are pregnant, breast feeding, have high blood pressure, diabetes, or kidney disease, consult your physician before taking *any* medication.

This table is based on information supplied by the manufacturers.

The second major category, narcotic painkillers, contains natural or artificial forms of opium. Common examples include codeine, propoxyphene (such as Darvon), meperidine (Demerol), and morphine. These drugs are often ordered to control short-term severe pain caused by cancer, surgery, or a fracture. Many prescription analgesics contain a combination of narcotic and nonnarcotic painkillers like acetaminophen and codeine (Tylenol with codeine and Tylox), aspirin with codeine (Empirin with codeine), propoxyphene and aspirin (Darvon Compound-65), and aspirin, caffeine, and butalibital (Fiorinal).

Narcotics should never be taken with alcohol, antihistamines, allergy or cold tablets, anticonvulsants, tranquilizers, muscle relaxants, or any other central nervous system (CNS) depressants. Life-threatening conditions can result from misuse or overdose.

CHAPTER REVIEW

Listing drugs:

Using Table 11-1, list example drug(s) in the following drug classifications. Do not list more than three in any one classification.

1. anesthetic: _____

_____

_____

_____

_____

2. corticosteroid: _____

_____

_____

_____

_____

3. emetic:_____

_____

_____

_____

_____

4. contraceptive: _____

_____

_____

_____

_____

5. vasoconstrictor: _____

_____

_____

_____

_____

6. antacid: _____

_____

_____

_____

_____

7. decongestant: _____

_____

_____

_____

_____

8. bronchodilator: _____

_____

_____

_____

_____

9. antiviral: _____

_____

_____

_____

_____

10. diuretic: _____

_____

_____

_____

_____

Listing drug classification:

Using text material, locate the following drugs and indicate which classification(s) they fall under.

11. Nupercaine _____

_____

_____

_____

_____

12. Sorbitrate _____

_____

_____

_____

_____

13. heparin _____

_____

_____

_____

14. Lomotil _____

_____

_____

_____

_____

15. Diamox _____

_____

_____

_____

_____

16. Topicort _____

_____

_____

_____

17. Gesterol _____

_____

_____

_____

_____

18. Pilocar ophthalmic solution _____

_____

_____

_____

_____

19. LSD _____

_____

_____

_____

_____

20. Mellaril _____

_____

_____

_____

_____

Appendices

Appendix A
Commonly Used Abbreviatons and Symbols

Abbreviations

A

A_2	aortic 2nd sound
AB	abortion
ABD; abd	abdominal
ABO	three main blood types
abbr	abbreviations
a.c.	before meals
ACh	acetylcholine
ACTH	adrenocorticotropic hormone
AD	right ear
ADH	antidiuretic hormone
ad lib	as desired
ADLs	activities of daily living
ADM	admission
AFB	acid-fast bacillus
AFP	alpha-fetoprotein
A/G	albumin-globulin ratio
Ag	silver
AJ	ankle jerk
AK	above knee
ALB; alb	albumin
ALKA PHOS; ALP	alkaline phosphatase
ALT	alanine aminotransferase (new for SGPT)
a.m.	antemeridian (midnight to noon)
AMA	against medical advice; American Medical Association
AMB; amb	ambulatory

AM J NURS	*American Journal of Nursing*
amp	ampere; ampule; amputation
amt	amount
ANA	antinuclear antibody
ANES	anesthesia
AP	anteroposterior
A&P; A/P	anterior and posterior; auscultation and percussion
AS	left ear
ASA	aspirin (acetylsalicylic acid)
ASAP	as soon as possible
ASOT	antistreptolysin O titer
AST	aspartateaminotransferase (new for SGOT)
AU	both ears
AV	arteriovenous
A-V; AV	atrioventricular

B

Ba	barium
BCP	blood chemistry profile
b.i.d.	twice a day
b.i.n.	twice a night
BK	below knee
BM	bowel movement
BMR	basal metabolic rate
BP	blood pressure
bpm	beats per minute
BPR	blood pressure; pulse; respiration
BR	bed rest
BRP	bathroom privileges
BS	blood sugar; breath sounds; bowel sounds
BUN	blood urea nitrogen
B&W	black and white
bx	biopsy

C

$\bar{c}$	with
C	carbon; Celsius (centigrade)
C1–C7	cervical vertebrae
C&S	culture and sensitivity
Ca	calcium; cancer; carcinoma
cal	calcium
CAT	computerized axial tomography
cath	catheter
CBC	complete blood count

CBR	complete bed rest
cc	cubic centimeter(s)
CC	chief complaint
CCU	coronary care unit
CHO	carbohydrate
chol	cholesterol
CK	creatine kinase
Cl	chloride
cl liq	clear liquid
cm	centimeter(s)
cmm	cubic millimeter(s)
CNS	central nervous system
c/o	complains of
CO	carbon monoxide compound
CO_2/CO2	carbon dioxide
cond	condition
cont	continue
CPK	creatine phosphokinase
CPR	cardiopulmonary resuscitation
CS	cesarean section
CSF	cerebrospinal fluid
CSR	central supply room
CV	cardiovascular; central venous
CVA	costovertebral angle; cerebrovascular accident
CVP	central venous pressure
cx	cervix
cxr	chest x-ray
cysto	cystoscopy

D

D1–12	dorsal (thoracic) vertebrae
db	decibel
D/C	discharge; discontinue
DC	Doctor of Chiropractic
D&C	dilatation and curettage
DAT	diet as tolerated
DDS	Doctor of Dental Surgery
DES	diethylstilbestrol
diff	differential
disch	discharge
DISP; disp	disposition
DNR	do not resuscitate
DO	Doctor of Osteopathy
DOA	dead on arrival

DOB	date of birth
DPT	diphtheria, pertussis, and tetanus
dr	dram, ʒ
Dr.	doctor
DRG	diagnosis related groups
DTR	deep tendon reflexes
DU	diagnosis undetermined
DX; dx	diagnosis

E

E. coli	Escherichia coli
ECC	electroconvulsive therapy
ECG	electrocardiogram
ECT	extra corporeal circulation
EENT	See *HEENT*
EEG	electroencephalogram
EKG	electrocardiogram
ELFD	elective low forceps delivery
ELIX; elix	elixir
EMG	electromyogram
ENT	ear, nose, and throat
EOMs	extraocular movements
epis	episiotomy
epith	epithelial
ERCP	endoscopic retrograde choleangiopancreatography
ESR	erythrocyte sedimentation rate
EST	electroshock therapy
etiol	etiology
ET	endotracheal
ETOH	ethyl alcohol
EUA	examined under anesthesia
exam	examination
exp	expended
ext	extended; extension; extraction; external; extremity

F

5-FU	5-Fluorouracil
F	Fahrenheit
FANA	fluorescent antinuclear antibody
FB	foreign body
FBS	fasting blood sugar
FDA	Food and Drug Administration
Fe	iron
FEV	forced expiratory volume

FH	family history; fetal head; fetal heart
FHR	fetal heart rate
FHS	fetal heart sounds
FHT	fetal heart tones
fl oz	fluid ounce
FR	French catheter (use only with a number)
FSH	follicle stimulating hormone
FTA-ABS	fluorescent treponemal Ab absorption test
FTT	failure to thrive
FUO	fever of undetermined origin
FVC	forced vital capacity
fx	fracture

G

g	gram
ga	gauge
GB	gallbladder
GI	gastrointestinal
GP	general practitioner
gr	grain
GRAV	gravida (number of times pregnant)
gtt	drop(s)
GTT	glucose tolerance test
GU	genitourinary
GYN; gyn	gynecology

H

H	hydrogen; hypodermic
H&H	hemoglobin and hematocrit
H&P	history and physical
HA	headache
HCG	human chorionic gonadotropin
HCl	hydrochloric acid
HCO_3	bicarbonate
Hct; hct	hematocrit
HDL	high density lipoproteins
HEENT	head, ears, eyes, nose, and throat
Hg	mercury
Hgb; hgb	hemoglobin
hGH	human growth hormone
HIV	human immunodeficiency virus
HOB	head of bed
HOSP	hospital
HPI	history of present illness
hr	hour

HR	heart rate
h.s.	hora somni; at bedtime
HSS	hot saline soaks
ht	height
HTLV-III	human T-cell lymphotropic virus
HX; hx	history
hypo	hypodermic

I

I	iodine
131–I; I131	radioactive iodine
I&D	incision and drainage
I&O	intake and output
IADH	inappropriate ADH
IC	intercostal; intracranial
ICP	intracranial pressure
ICS	intercostal space
ICU	intensive care unit
ID	identification
IgA; IgD; IgE; IgG; IgM	immunoglobins
IM	intramuscular
IMP	impression
INHAL	inhalation
INJ	inject; injection
INSTR	instruction
IP	interphalangeal
IPPB	intermittent positive pressure breathing
IQ; I.Q.	intelligence quotient
isol	isolation
IU	immunization unit
IUD	intrauterine device
IV	intravenous
IVC	intravenous cholangiogram
IVP	intravenous pyelogram

J

JAMA	*Journal of the American Medical Association*
JCAHO	Joint Commission on Accreditation of Healthcare Organizations
JVD	jugular vein distention

K

K+	potassium
KCl	potassium chloride

kg	kilogram
KI	potassium iodide
KLS	kidney, liver, spleen
KUB	kidney, ureters, bladder

L

L; l	liter
L1–L5	lumbar vertebrae
L & A	light and accommodation
L & D	labor and delivery
L & W	living and well
lac	laceration
LAD	left anterior decending
lap	laparotomy
lat	lateral
LCCA	left common carotid artery
LD; LDH	lactic dehydrogenase
LDL	low density lipoproteins
L/E	lower extremity
LE cell	lupus erythematosus cell
LFT	liver function test
LH	luteinizing hormone
LKS	liver, kidneys, spleen
LLE	left lower extremity
LLL	left lower lobe
LLQ	left lower quadrant
LMP	last menstrual period
LNMP	last normal menstrual period
LOA; loa	leave of absence
LOC	level of consciousness
LoNa	low sodium
LP	lumbar puncture
LPN	licensed practical nurse
LUL	left upper lobe
LUQ	left upper quadrant

M

m	meter; minim (equivalent to a drop)
M1	mitral first heart sound
MAP	mean arterial pressure
MAR	Medication Administration Record
max	maximum
mc	millicurie
mcg	microgram

MCH	mean corpuscular cell hemoglobin
MCHC	mean corpuscular hemoglobin concentration
MCV	mean corpuscular volume
MED	medical; medicine
mEq	milliequivalent
mets	metastases
mg	milligram
Mg	magnesium
MH	marital history
min	minute; minimum
ml	milliliter
mm	millimeter
mmHg	millimeter of mercury
mmol	millimoles
MOPP	nitrogen mustard, oncovin, prednisone, procarbazine
MRI	magnetic resonance imaging
ms	morphine sulfate

N

N	nitrogen
N_2O; N2O	nitrous oxide
Na	sodium
NA	nurse's assistant
NaCl	sodium chloride (salt)
NAS	no added salt
NB	newborn
NCD	not considered disqualifying
nec	not elsewhere classified
NEG	negative
NEURO	neurology
NG	nasogastric
NICU	neurological intensive care unit
NIS	not in stock
NKA	no known allergies
NNP	no nocturnal paroxysms
NOC; noc; noct	nocturnal
NPH	neutral protein Hagedorn (insulin)
NPN	nonprotein nitrogen
n.p.o.	nothing by mouth
NSO	Nursing Service Office
NSR	normal sinus rhythm
nsy	nursery
NT	nasotracheal
N & V	nausea and vomiting
NWB	no weightbearing

O

O_2; O2	oxygen
OB	obstetrics
OCG	oral cholecystogram
OD	right eye; overdose; Doctor of Optometry
oint	ointment
OOB	out of bed
OR	operating room
ORTHO	orthopedics
OS	left eye
OT	occupational therapy
OTR	registered occupational therapist
OU	both eyes
oz	ounce

P

$\bar{p}$	after
P	phosphorus; pulse
P_2; P2	pulmonic second sound
PA	physician's assistant; posteroanterior
PACU	post anesthesic care unit
PA&LAT	posteroanterior and lateral
P&A	percussion and auscultation
PAL	prisoner at large
Pap	Papanicolaou (smear)
para	number of liveborns delivered
PBI	protein-bound iodine
p.c.	after meals
pCO_2; pCO2	carbon dioxide pressure
PCV	packed cell volume
PDR	*Physician's Desk Reference*
PE	physical examination
PEDS; Peds	pediatrics
PEEP	positive end expiratory pressure
PEG	pneumoencephalogram
Pent	Pentothal
per	through; by means of
PERLA/PERRLA	pupils equal, round, and react to light and accommodation
PET	positron-emission tomography
PhD	Doctor of Philosophy
pH (symbol)	hydrogen ion concentration
PH	past history; personal history; public health
PHN	Public Health Nurse

PHR	pharmacy
PI	present illness
PICU	Peds Intensive Care Unit
PIP	proximal interphalangeal
PKU	phenylketonuria
p.m.	post meridian, between noon and midnight; postmortem
PMI	point of maximum impulse
PMNs	polymorphonuclear leukocytes
PNS	peripheral nervous system
p.o.	by mouth (orally)
PO	phone order; postoperative
POD	postoperative day
PP	postprandial; postpartum
PPBS	postprandial blood sugar
PPD	purified protein derivative
PPM	parts per million
pr	pair
PR	pulse rate; packed red blood cells
PRE	passive resistance exercises
PREG	pregnant
PREOP	preoperative
PREP	prepare
p.r.n.	pro re nata; when necessary; as needed
PRO	prothrombin time
PROM	premature rupture of membrane; passive range of motion
PSP	phenolsulfonphthalein
pt	patient; pint
PT	prothrombin time; physical therapy
PTH	parathyroid hormone
PTT	partial thromboplastin test or time
PUD	pregnancy, uterine, delivered
PUND	pregnancy, uterine, not delivered
PWB	partial weight bearing

Q

q suff	as much as will suffice
Q; q	every
q.a.m.	every morning
qd	every day
qh	every hour
q2h	every 2 hours
q3h	every 3 hours
q4h	every 4 hours

q6h	every 6 hours
q8h	every 8 hours
q.i.d.	four times a day
qn	every night
QNS	quantity not sufficient
q.o.d.	every other day
qoh	every other hour
q.p.	as much as desired
q p.m.	every evening
QS	quantity sufficient
qt	quart
qual	quality; qualitative
quant	quantity; quantitative

R

R	right; rectal; respiration
R/O	rule out
Ra	radium
rbc	red blood cell
RBC	red blood count
REM	rapid eye movement
RESP	respirator; respiratory
RF	rheumatoid factor
Rh	Rhesus factor
RLL	right lower lobe
RLQ	right lower quadrant
R&M	routine and microscopic
RML	right middle lobe
RN	registered nurse
ROM	range of motion
ROS	review of systems
RR	recovery room
RSR	regular sinus rhythm
rt	right
RT	respiratory therapy
RUL	right upper lobe
RUQ	right upper quadrant
Rx	prescription

S

$\bar{s}$	without
S	sulfur
S1–S5	sacral vertebrae
SA; S-A	sinoatrial (node)

S&A	sugar and acetone
SGD	straight gravity drainage
SGOT	serum glutamic oxaloacetic transaminase
SGPT	serum glutamic pyruvic transaminase
SH	social history
SICU	Surgical Intensive Care Unit
SOB	short of breath
SOL	solution
s.o.s.	if necessary
S/P	status post
SP GR; Sp Gr	specific gravity
SR	sedimentation rate
ss	one-half
S/S	signs and symptoms
SSE	soap suds enema
staph	staphylococcus
STAT; stat	immediately
strep	streptococcus
STS	serological test for syphilis
STSG	split thickness skin graft
sub ling	under tongue
sub-Q	subcutaneous
SUPP; supp	suppository
SURG	surgical
SUSP	suspension
SYR	syrup
sx	symptoms

T

T1–T12	thoracic vertebrae
T	temperature
T_3	one thyroid function test
T_4	one thyroid function test
tab	tablet
tsp	teaspoonful
tbsp	tablespoonful
Tc; 99uTc	technetium
TCT	thrombin clotting time
ther	therapy
t.i.d.	three times a day
tinct	tincture
TLC	tender loving care
TM	tympanic membrane
TNM	tumor, nodes, metastases

TO	telephone order
TP	total protein
TPN	total parenteral nutrition
TPR	temperature, pulse, and respiration
TWE	tap water enema
T&X-match	type and crossmatch
tx	treatment

U

U	unit
UA	urinalysis
UCD; UCHD	usual childhood diseases
μg	microgram
UGI	upper gastrointestinal
UNG; ung	ointment
U/O	urine output
UVL	ultraviolet light

V

VA	Veterans Administration
VAG; vag	vagina; vaginal
VC	vital capacity
VD	venereal disease
VDRL	Venereal Disease Research Laboratories
VO	verbal order
VPRC	volume of packed red cells
VS	vital signs

W

w/c	wheelchair
wbc	white blood cell
WBC	white blood count
WD	well-developed
WDWN; w/d w/n	well-developed, well-nourished
WNL	within normal limits
WO	without
wt	weight
W/V	weight per volume

X

X; x	multiplied by; by; times

Y

YO	year old
YOB	year of birth

Z

Zn	zinc

SYMBOLS

Ⓛ	left	↑	elevation
Ⓡ	right	↑	increased
♂	male	♀	female
°	degree	′	foot
#	weight, gauge, number	24°	24 hours
″	inch	?	question of
+	plus; positive	2°	secondary
−	negative; minus	1 ×	once
?	questionable	× 2	two times
2 ×	twice	>	greater than
↓	decreased	▲	change
↓	depression		
<	less than		

Appendix B
Medical Terminology Elements

Element	Meaning
a-	without; not
-a/sthenia	weakness (not strong)
ab-	away from; not
acoust(i)-	hearing; sound
acro-	extremities
aden-	gland
adnexa	ties; connections
adreno-	adrenal gland
aer-	air
-algia	pain
alveol-	cavity; socket
ambi-	both
ameb-	change
amphi-	around; on both sides
an-	without; not
angi-	vessels (usually blood)
ante-	before
anti-	against
antr-	cavity or chamber
apo-	away from
appendic-	appendix
arter-	artery
arthr-	joint
astr-	star shaped
aur-	ear
auto-	self
basi-	base; bottom part
benign	not cancerous

bi-	two; double; both
bili-	bile
blast-	bud; immature
blephar-	eyelids
brachy-	short
brady-	slow
bronch-	bronchus
bucc(o)-	cheek
burso-	sac
calc-	heel; stone
cantho-	angle at the end of the eyelid
capit-	head
carcin-	cancer
cardi-	heart
cata-	down
cauda-	tail
cauter-	burn
cec-	blind passage; cecum
-cele	hernia; tumor; swelling
celio-	abdomen
-centesis	puncture
cephal-	head
cerebr-	brain
cervic-	cervix
cheil-	lip
cheir-	hand
chir-	hand
chole-	bile; gall
chondr-	cartilage
cilia	eyelash
cine-	move; movement
-clast	break
col-	colon
colla-	glue; gelatin-like
colp(o)-	hollow; vagina
contra-	against; counter
cor	heart
corne-	horny; horn-like
cost-	rib
crani-	skull
-crine	to secrete
cryo-	cold
cut-	skin
cyan-	blue
cyst	noun: sac containing fluid element: bladder

cyt-	cell
dacry-	tear
dactyl-	finger; toe
dendr-	tree; branching (usually nervous system)
dent-	teeth
dermat-	skin
-desis	binding; fixation
di-	twice
dia-	through
digit	finger; toe
dis-	apart
dors-	back
duct-	tube; draw; lead
duodeno-	duodenum
dura	hard
dynam-	power; force
-dynia	pain
dys-	bad; out of order
-e	instrument
-ectasis	expansion
-ectomy	surgical removal of all or part of
edema-	swelling by fluid
-emesis	vomiting
en-	in
encephal-	brain
end-	inside; within
enter-	intestines (usually small)
ependym-	wrapping; a covering
epi-	upon; in addition to
erythro-	red
esophag-	esophagus
-esthesia	sensation; feeling
eu-	good
eury-	broad
ex-	out; away from
fac-	make; do
fascia	sheet; band
fiss-	split
fistul-	pipe; a narrow passage
furca-	fork-shaped
gangli-	swelling; knot-like mass
gastr-	stomach
gen-	original; production
ger-	old
gingiv-	gum

glom-	ball; mass
glosso-	tongue
glyco-	sweet; sugar
grad-	walk; take steps
-gram	record; write
gran-	grain; particle
gravid	pregnant
gyn-	female
hallux-	great toe
helio-	sun; light
hem(at)-	blood
hemi-	half
hepat-	liver
heter-	other
histo-	tissue
hom-	same
hormone	to excite or set in motion
hydro-	water
hyper-	above; more than normal
hypno-	sleep
hypo-	under; beneath; deficient
hyster-	uterus
-iasis	formation of; presence of
ile-	ileum
ili-	ilium
infer-	under; below
infra-	beneath
inter-	between
intra-	within
iris	colored eye membrane
iso-	equal
-itis	inflammation
kerat-	horny tissue
labi-	lip
lacrim-	tear
lact-	milk
lal-	speech
lapar-	abdominal wall
laryng-	larynx
later-	side
leio-	smooth
lept-	slender
leuk-	white
lien-	spleen
lig-	ligament

lingua-	language; speech
lip-	fat
lith-	stone
lobo-	section
lumbo-	loins
lymph-	watery fluid
-lysis	loosening; destruction
macro-	large
macul-	spot or stain
mal-	bad
-malacia	soft condition
malign-	cancerous
mamm-	breast
mani-	mental disturbance
mast-	breast
maxill-	upper jawbone
mechano-	machine
med-	middle
-megaly	enlarged
melan-	black
mening-	membrane
ment-	mind
meta-	beyond; change
metabol(e)-	change
metr-	uterus
mi-	less; smaller
micr-	small
morph-	form
my-	muscle
myco-	fungus
myel-	bone marrow; spinal cord
myring-	eardrum
necr-	dead
neo-	new
nephr-	kidney
neuro-	nerve or nervous system
ocul-	eye
odont-	tooth
-oid	like; resembling
olfact-	smell
-ologist	a specialist
-ology	study of
-oma	tumor
oment-	covering of abdominal organs
onco-	mass; tumor; swelling

onych-	nail; claw
oophor-	ovary
ophthalm-	eye (diagnostic)
opt-	eye (anatomical)
or-	mouth
orchi-	testis
orth-	straight
-osis	condition (usually excessive)
osmo-	odor
ost(eo)-	bone
-ostomy	to create an opening
oto-	ear
-otomy	incision
ovar-	ovary; egg
ovario-	ovary
pachy-	thick
palpebr-	eyelid
pan-	all
para-	beside; beyond
pariet-	wall
part-	labor
path-	disease
pect-	chest
pelvis	pelvis
-penia	decrease
peps-	digest
per-	throughout
peri-	about; around
-pexy	suspension; fixation
phage	to eat
phak-	lens
pharmac-	drug
pharyng-	pharynx
phleb-	vein
phob-	fear
phon-	voice; sound
phot-	light
phrag-	fence; wall off
phren-	mind
physio-	function
pilo-	hair
plak-	plate; lens
plasia-	development; growth
plast-	plastic repair
platy-	flat; plate; broad

-plegia	paralysis
plexus	braid; network
pneum-	lung; air
pod-	foot
poly-	many; much
post	after; behind in time
poster-	back part
pre-	in front of; before
pro-	in front of; before
proct-	anus
proli-	offspring; production
proxim-	nearest
pseud-	false
psycho-	mind
-ptosis	falling; drooping
ptyal-	saliva
puer-	child
pulmon-	lung
pyle	gate
pyloro-	pylorus
rachi-	spinal column
radi-	ray
radic-	root
ramus	branch
ren-	kidney
retr(o)-	backwards
rhin-	nose
-rrhag	burst
-rrhaphy	suture
-rrhea	flow
-rrhexis	burst; rupture
rug-	wrinkle; fold; crease
sacro-	sacrum
salpingo-	tube (usually fallopian)
sarc-	flesh
schiz-	split
scirr(h)-	hard
scler(a)-	hard
scol-	curved
-scop	look; observe
sedat-	quiet; calm
semen	male reproductive fluid
semi-	half
sept-	wall; fence
sinus	hollow space

somato-	body
somni-	sleep
spas-	pull; draw
spasm	involuntary contractions
sphenic-	wedge-shaped
spiro-	coil
splen-	spleen
spondyl-	spinal column or vertebra
squam-	scale
sta-	stand
steno-	narrow; contracted
stoma-	mouth or opening
strept-	twist
strict-	to draw tight; narrowing
sub-	under; beneath; below
supra-	above; over
sym-	together
syn-	together
tarso-	framework of the upper eyelid; ankle region; instep
tegument	skin; covering
tens-	stretch
thalam-	inner chamber
thel-	nipple
therap-	therapy
therm-	heat
thorac-	chest
thromb-	lump; clot
thyro-	thyroid
ton-	stretch
-tope	place
trachel-	neck; neckline structure
trans-	through; across
traumat-	wound; injury
tri-	three
trich-	hair
trip-	rub; friction
-trophy	development; growth
tumor	swelling
turbin-	shaped like a top
tympan-	eardrum; eardrum enclosure
umbilic-	navel
ureter	ureter
urethra	urethra
utero-	uterus
vaso-	vessel

vena-	vein
ventr-	front
vert-	turn
vesic-	bladder (anatomical)
vestibule	entrance
viscero-	organ
volv-	roll; turn
vuls(e)-	twitch; pull
xer-	dry

Appendix C
Commonly Prescribed Drugs

Brand Name	Manufacturer	Generic Name
Trimox	Apothecon	amoxicillin
Premarin	Wyeth-Ayerst	conjugated estrogens
Synthroid	Knoll	levothyroxine
Hydrocodone w/APAP	Watson	hydrocodone w/APAP
Prozac	Dista	fluoxetine
Lanoxin	Glaxo Wellcome	digoxin
Prilosec	Astra/Merck	omeprazole
Vasotec	Merck & Co.	enalapril
Zithromax	Pfizer	azithromycin
Norvasc	Pfizer	amlodipine
Zoloft	Pfizer	sertraline
Claritin	Schering	loratadine
Coumadin	Du Pont Pharm	warfarin
Augmentin	SmithKline Beecham	amoxicillin/ clavulanate
Zocor	Merck	simvastatin
Furosemide	Mylan	furosemide
Paxil	SmithKline Beecham	paroxetine
Albuterol Aerosol	Warrick	albuterol
Zantac	Glaxo/Wellcome	ranitidine
Zestril	Zeneca Pharm	lisinopril
Procardia XL	Pfizer	nifedipine
Prempro	Wyeth-Ayerst	conj.estrogens/ medroxy- progesterone
Cardizem CD	Hoechst Marion R	diltiazem
Biaxin	Abbott	clarithromycin

Brand Name	Manufacturer	Generic Name
Amoxil	SmithKline Beecham	amoxicillin
Trimeth/Sulfameth	Teva	trimeth/sulfameth
Cephalexin	Teva	cephalexin
Acetaminophen/ Codeine	Teva	acetaminophen/ codeine
Glucophage	Bristol-Myers/Squibb	metformin
Cipro	Bayer Pharm	ciprofloxacin
Propoxyphene N/APAP	Mylan	propoxyphene N/APAP
Veetids	Apothecon	penicillin VK
Amoxicillin	Teva	amoxicillin
Pravachol	Bristol-Myers Squibb	pravastatin
Triamterene/HCTZ	Geneva	triamterene/HCTZ
Ultram	McNeil	tamadol
Hytrin	Abbott	terazosin
Ambien	Searle	zolpidem
Levoxyl	Daniels	levothyroxine
Ortho-Novum 7/7/7	Ortho Pharm	norethindrone/ethinyl estradiol
K-Dur-20	Schering	potassium chloride
Accupril	Parke-Davis	quinapril
Triphasil	Wyeth-Ayerst	L-norgestrel/ethinyl estradiol
Relafen	SmithKline Beecham	nabumetone
Amitriptyline	Mylan	amitriptyline
Claritin D 12HR	Schering	loratidine/ pseudoephedrine
Humulin N	Lilly	human insulin-NPH
Dilantin	Parke-Davis	phenytoin
Pepcid	Merck & Co	famotidine
Glucotrol XL	Pfizer	glipizide
Lotensin	Novartis	benazepril
Prinivil	Merck & Co	lisinopril
Cephalexin	Apothecon	cephalexin
Acetaminophen/ Codeine	Purepac	acetaminophen/ codeine
Cardura	Pfizer	doxazosin
Mevacor	Merck & Co	lovastatin
Cefzil	Bristol-Myers Squibb	cefprozil
Xanax	Pharmacia & UpJohn	alprazolam
Prednisone	Schein	prednisone
Atenolol	Mylan	atenolol
Lipitor	Parke-Davis	atorvastatin
Propulsid	Janssen	cisapride

Brand Name	Manufacturer	Generic Name
Lorazepam	Mylan	lorazepam
Diflucan	Pfizer	fluconazole
Atrovent	Boehringer Ingelheim	ipratropium
Depakote	Abbott	divalproex
Adalat CC	Bayer Pharm	nifedipine
Prevacid	Tap Pharm	lansoprazole
Glyburide	Copley	glyburide
Ceftin	Glaxo Wellcome	cefuroxime
Toprol-XL	Astra	metoprolol
Propoxyphene N/APAP	Teva	propoxyphene N/APAP
Pondimin	Wyeth Ayerst	fenfluramine
Zyrtec	Pfizer	cetirizine
Lescol	Novartis	fluvastatin
Daypro	Searle	oxaprozin
Ortho Tri-Cyclen	Ortho Pharm	norgestimate/ ethinyl estradiol
Albuterol Neb Soln	Warrick	albuterol
Flonase	Glaxo Wellcome	fluticasone
Ery-Tab	Abbott	erythromycin
Imdur	Schering	isosorbide mononitrate S.A.
Verapamil SR	Zenith	verapamil
Imitrex	Glaxo Wellcome	sumatriptan
Nitrostat	Parke-Davis	nitroglycerin
Clonazepam	Teva	clonazepam
Cycrin	ESI Lederle	medroxyprogesterone
BuSpar	Bristol-Myers Squibb	buspirone
Allegra	Hoech Mar R	fexofenadine
Humulin 70/30	Lilly	human insulin 70/30
Axid	Lilly	nizatidine
Vancenase AQ DS	Schering	beclomethasone
Atenolol	ESI Lederle	atenolol
Lotrisone	Schering	clotrimoxazole/ betamethasone
Naprosyn	Syntax	naproxen
Hydrocodone/APAP	Qualitest	hydrocodone/APAP
Phentermine	Eon Labs	phentermine
Lorazepam	Purepac	lorazepam
Cozaar	Merck & Co	losartan
Azmacort	Hoech Mar R	triamcinolone aerosol
Fosamax	Merck & Co	alendronate
Desogen	Organon	desogestrel/ ethinyl estradiol

Brand Name	Manufacturer	Generic Name
Alprazolam	Greenstone	alprazolam
Lo/Ovral	Wyeth-Ayerst	norgestrel/ ethinyl estradiol
Roxicet	Roxane	oxycodone/APAP
Albuterol Aerosol	Zenith	albuterol
Proventil Aerosol	Schering	albuterol
Atenolol	Geneva	atenolol
Metoprolol Tartrate	Mylan	metoprolol
Klor-Con	Upsher-Smith	potassium chloride
Medroxy- progesterone	Greenstone	medroxyprogesterone
Serevent	Glaxo Wellcome	salmeterol
Cyclobenzaprine	Mylan	cyclobenzaprine
Deltasone	Pharmacia/Upjohn	prednisone
Methylphenidate	M.D. Pharm	methylphenidate
Triamterene/HCTZ	Mylan	triamterene/HCTZ
Provera	Pharmacia/Upjohn	medroxyprogesterone
Monopril	Bristol-Myers Squibb	fosinopril
Tri-Levlen	Berlex	L-norgestrel/ethinyl estradiol
Ziac	Wyeth-Ayerest	bisoprolol/HCTZ
Neomycin/ Polymx/HC	Schein	neomycin/polymx/HC
Carisoprodol	Schein	carisoprodol
Estrace	Bristol-Myers Squibb	estradiol
Ortho-Cyclen	Ortho Pharm	norgestimate/ethinyl estradiol
Ibuprofen	Par Pharm	ibuprofen
Diazepam	Mylan	diazepam
Macrobid	Procter & Gamble	nitrofurantoin
Ortho-Cept	Ortho Pharm	desogestrel/ethinyl estradiol
Bactroban	SmithKline Beecham	mupirocin
Cimetidine	Mylan	cimetidine
Claritin D 24HR	Schering	loratidine/ pseudoephedrine
Effexor	Wyeth-Ayerst	venlafaxine
Methylprednisolone	Duramed Ph	methylprednisolone
Loestrin-FE 1.5/30	Parke-Davis	norethindrone/ ethinyl estradiol
Redux	Wyeth-Ayerst	dexfenfluramine
Guaifenesin/PPA	Duramed	guaifenesin/phenyl- propanolamine
Risperdal	Janssen	risperidone
Cefaclor	Mylan	cefaclor

Brand Name	Manufacturer	Generic Name
Temazepam	Mylan	temazepam
Glyburide	Greenstone	glyburide
Lorabid	Lilly	loracarbef
Propacet 100	Teva	propoxyphene N/APAP
Endocet	Endo Gen Pd	oxycodone/APAP
Retin-A	Ortho Derm	tretinoin
Calan SR	Searle	verapamil
Alprazolam	Mylan	alprazolam
Gemfibrozil	Warner Chiloott	gemfibrozil
Potassium Chloride	Ethex	potassium chloride
Lasix	Hoech Mar R	furosemide
Atenolol	Apothecon	atenolol
Phenergan Supp	Wyeth-Ayerst	promethazine
Lodine	Wyeth-Ayerst	etodolac
Dyazide	SmithKline Beecham	hydrochlorothiazide/ triamterine
Xalatan	Pharmacia/Upjohn	latanoprost
Glipizide	Mylan	glipizide
Clonidine	Mylan	clonidine
Naproxen	Teva	naproxen
Hydrocodone w/APAP	Mallinckrdt	hydrocodone w/APAP
Humulin R	Lilly	human insulin regular
Floxin	Ortho Pharm	ofloxacin
Ventolin Aerosol	Glaxo Wellcome	albuterol
Vanceril	Schering	beclomethasone
Zovirax	Glaxo Wellcome	acyclovir
Glynase Prestab	Pharmacia/Upjohn	glyburide
Estradiol	Watson	estradiol
Guaifenesin/PPA	Sidmak	guaifenesin/phenyl- propanolamine
Doxycycline	Zenith	doxycycline
Elocon	Schering	mometasone
Alprazolam	Purepac	alprazolam
Serzone	Bristol-Myers Squibb	nefazodone
Zestoretic	Zeneca Pharm	lisinopril/HCTZ
Loestrin-Fe 1/20	Parke-Davis	Norethindrone/ ethinyl estradiol
Furosemide	Watson	furosemide
Ibu	Knoll	ibuprofen
Trusopt	Merck & Co	dorzolamide
Tobradex	Alcon Lab	tobramycin/ dexamethasone

Brand Name	Manufacturer	Generic Name
Altace	Hoechst Marion Roussel	ramipril
Darvocet-N 100	Lilly	propoxyphene-N/APAP
Cyclobenzaprine	Schein	cyclobenzaprine
Dicyclomine	Rugby	dicyclomine
Hydrochlorothiazide	ESI Lederle	hydrochlorothiazide
Metoprolol Tartrate	Geneva	metoprolol
Amoxicillin	Warner-Chilcott	amoxicillin
Promethazine/ Codeine	Barre	promethazine/ Codeine
Klonopin	Roche	clonazepam
Ortho-Novum 1/35	Ortho Pharm	norethindrone/ ethinyl estradiol
Trazodone	Sidmak	trazodone
Neurontin	Parke-Davis	gabapentin
Nitro-Dur	Schering	nitroglycerin
Tamoxifen	Barr	tamoxifen
Biaxin Susp	Abbott	clarithromycin
Rhinocort	Astra USA	budesonide
Estraderm	Novartis	estradiol
Genora 1/35	Rugby	norethindrone/ ethinyl estradiol
Suprax	Wyeth-Ayerst	cefixime
Xanax	Pharmacia/Upjohn	alprazolam
Timoptic XE	Merck & Co	timolol
Demulen 1/35	Searle	ethynodiol/ ethinyl estradiol
Albuterol Oral Liq	Warrick	albuterol

Appendix D
Look-Alike Sound-Alike Drugs

Accubron	Accutane
Accutane	Accubron
Accutane	Acutrim
acetazolamide	acetohexamide
acetohexamide	acetazolamide
Achromycin	actinomycin C
Achromycin	Adriamycin
Actidil	Actifed
Actifed	Actidil
actinomycin C	Achromycin
Acutrim	Accutane
Adapin	Adapt
Adapin	Atabrine
Adapt	Adapin
Adriamycin	Achromycin
Adriamycin	Idamycin
Afrin	Arfonad
Afrin	aspirin
Agoral	Argyrol
Akineton	Ecotrin
Albutein	albuterol
albuterol	Albutein
Aldactazide	Aldactone
Aldactone	Aldactazide
Aldomet	Aldoril
Aldoril	Aldomet
Aldoril	Elavil
alfentanil	Anafranil
alfentanil	fentanyl

alfentanil	sufentanil
alprazolam	lorazepam
Altace	alteplase
alteplase	Altace
alteplase	anistreplase
Alupent	Atrovent
Amcill	Amoxil
Amicar	Amikin
Amikin	Amicar
aminophylline	amitriptyline
aminophylline	ampicillin
amiodarone	amrinone
Amipaque	Omnipaque
amitriptyline	aminophylline
amoxacillin	amoxapine
amoxapine	amoxacillin
amoxapine	Amoxil
Amoxil	Amcill
Amoxil	amoxapine
ampicillin	aminophylline
amrinone	amiodarone
Anafranil	alfentail
Anaprox	Anaspaz
Anaspaz	Anaprox
anisindione	anistropine
anistreplase	alteplase
anistropine	anisindione
Ansaid	Axsain
Antabuse	Anturane
Anturane	Antabuse
Anturane	Artane
Anusol	Aquasol
Aplisol	Aplitest
Aplitest	Aplisol
Apresazide	Apresoline
Apresoline	Apresazide
Apresoline	Priscoline
Aquasol	Anusol
Aralen	Arlidin
Arfonad	Afrin
Argyrol	Agoral
Arlidin	Aralen
Artane	Anturane
aspirin	Afrin
Atabrine	Adapin

Atabrine	Ativan
Atarax	Ativan
atenolol	timolol
Ativan	Atabrine
Ativan	Atarax
Ativan	Avitene
Atrovent	Alupent
Avitene	Ativan
Axsain	Ansaid
azatadine	azathioprine
azathioprine	azatadine
azathioprine	azidothymidine
azathioprine	Azulfidine
azidothymidine	azathioprine
Azlin	Mezlin
Azulfidine	azathioprine
bacitracin	Bactrim
bacitracin	Bactroban
baclofen	Beclovent
Bactine	Bactrim
Bactocill	Pathocil
Bactrim	bacitracin
Bactrim	Bactine
Bactroban	bacitracin
Banthine	Brethine
Beclovent	baclofen
Benadryl	Bentyl
Benadryl	Benylin
Benadryl	Caladryl
Benoxyl	Brevoxyl
Bentyl	Benadryl
Bentyl	Bontril
Benylin	Benadryl
Benylin	Ventolin
benztropine	bromocriptine
Bicillin	V-Cillin
Brontril	Bentyl
Brontril	Vontrol
Brethaire	Brethine
Brethaire	Bretylol
Brethine	Banthine
Brethine	Brethaire
Bretylol	Brethaire
Bretylol	Brevital
Brevital	Bretylol

Brevoxyl	Benoxyl
bromocriptine	benztropine
Bumex	Buprenex
bupivacaine	mepivacaine
Buprenex	Bumex
bupropion	buspirone
buspirone	bupropion
butabarbital	Butalbital
Butalbital	butabarbital
Butazolidin	Butisol
Butisol	Butazolidin
Cafergot	Carafate
Caladryl	Benadryl
Caladryl	calamine
calamine	Caladryl
calciferol	calcitriol
calcitonin	calcitriol
calcitriol	calciferol
calcitriol	calcitonin
calcium glubionate	calcium gluconate
calcium gluconate	calcium glubionate
Cankaid	Enkaid
Capastat	Capastat
Capitrol	Captopril
Captopril	Capitrol
Carafate	Cafergot
Cardene	codeine
Cardilate	Cardiolite
Cardiolite	Cardilate
Cardura	cordarone
Catapres	Catarase
Catapres	Cetapred
Catapres	Combipres
Catapres	Diupres
Catarase	Catapres
cefamandole	cefmetazole
cefazolin	cephalothin
cefmetazole	cefamandole
Cefobid	cefonicid
cefonicid	Cefobid
Cefotan	Ceftin
cefotaxime	cefoxitin
cefotaxime	cefuroxime
cefoxitin	cefotaxime
cefoxitin	Cytoxan

ceftazidime	ceftizoxime
Ceftin	Cefotan
ceftizoxime	ceftazidime
cefuroxime	cefotaxime
Centoxin	Cytoxan
Centrax	Centrum
Centrum	Centrax
Cepastat	Capastat
cephalexin	cephalothin
cephalothin	cefazolin
cephalothin	cephalexin
cephapirin	cephradine
cephradine	cephapirin
Ceptaz	Septra
Cetaphil	Cetapred
Cetapred	Catapres
Cetapred	Cetaphil
Chenix	Chymex
Chlor-Trimeton	Chloromycetin
Chloromycetin	Chlor-Trimeton
chlorpromazine	chlorpropamide
chlorpromazine	promethazine
chlorpropamide	chlorpromazine
Chorex	Chymex
Chymex	Chenix
Chymex	Chorex
Chymex	Cystex
Cidex	Lidex
Ciloxan	Cytoxan
cimetidine	simethicone
Citracal	Citrucel
Citrucel	Citracal
Cleocin	Clinoril
Cleocin	Lincocin
Clinoril	Cleocin
clofazimine	clonazepam
clofazimine	clozapine
Clomid	clonidine
clomiphene	clomipramine
clomiphene	clonidine
clomipramine	clomiphene
clonazepam	clofazimine
clonidine	Clomid
clonidine	clomiphene
clonidine	Klonopin

clonidine	quinidine
clotrimazole	co-trimoxazole
clozapine	clofazimine
co-trimoxazole	clotrimazole
codeine	Cardene
codeine	Cordran
codeine	Lodine
Colestid	colistin
colestipol	colistin
colistin	Colestid
colistin	colestipol
Combipres	Catapres
cordarone	Cardura
cordarone	Cordran
Cordran	codeine
Cordran	cordarone
Cort-Dome	Cortone
Cortone	Cort-Dome
Coumadin	Kemadrin
cyclobenzaprine	cycloserine
cyclobenzaprine	cyproheptadine
cycloserine	cyclobenzaprine
cycloserine	cyclosporine
Cyclospasmol	cyclosporin
cyclosporin	Cyclospasmol
cyclosporin	Cyklokapron
cyclosporine	cycloserine
Cyklokapron	cyclosporin
cyproheptadine	cyclobenzaprine
Cystex	Chymex
Cytoxan	cefoxitin
Cytoxan	Centoxin
Cytoxan	Ciloxan
dacarbazine	Dicarbosil
Dacriose	Danocrine
Dalmane	Demulen
Danocrine	Dacriose
Daranide	Daraprim
Daraprim	Daranide
Daricon	Darvon
Darvocet-N	Darvon-N
Darvon	Daricon
Darvon-N	Darvocet-N
Demerol	Demulen
Demerol	Deprol

Demerol	Dymelor
Demerol	Temaril
Demulen	Dalmane
Demulen	Demerol
Depen	Endep
Deprol	Demerol
deserpidine	desipramine
Desferal	Disophrol
desipramine	deserpidine
desipramine	disopyramide
desipramine	imipramine
desoximetasone	dexamethasone
Desoxyn	digitoxin
Desoxyn	digoxin
Desyrel	Zestril
dexamethasone	desoximetasone
Dexedrine	Dextran
Dexedrine	Excedrin
Dextran	Dexedrine
Diamox	Trimox
diazepam	diazoxide
diazoxide	diazepam
diazoxide	Dyazide
Dicarbosil	dacarbazine
dichlorecetic acid	trichloracetic acid
diclofenac	Diflucan
dicylomine	dyclonine
Diflucan	diclofenac
digitoxin	Desoxyn
digitoxin	digoxin
digoxin	Desoxyn
digoxin	digitoxin
Dilantin	Dilaudid
Dilantin	diltiazem
Dilaudid	Dilantin
diltiazem	Dilantin
Dimetane	Dimetapp
Dimetapp	Dimetane
dipyridamole	disopyramide
Disophrol	Desferal
Disophrol	Stilphostrol
disopyramide	desipramine
disopyramide	dipyridamole
dithranol	Ditropan
Ditropan	dithranol

Ditropan	Intropin
Diupres	Catapres
Diupres	Diurese
Diupres	Hydropres
Diurese	Diupres
dobutamine	dopamine
Donnagel	Donnatal
Donnatal	Donnagel
dopamine	dobutamine
doxacurium	doxorubicin
doxapram	doxazocin
doxapram	doxepin
doxapram	Doxinate
doxazocin	doxapram
doxazocin	doxarubicin
doxazocin	doxepin
doxepin	doxapram
doxepin	doxazocin
doxepin	Doxidan
Doxidan	doxepin
Doxinate	doxapram
doxorubicin	doxacurium
doxorubicin	doxazocin
doxycycline	doxylamine
doxylamine	doxycycline
dronabinol	droperidol
droperidol	dronabinol
Dyazide	diazoxide
Dyazide	Thiacide
dyclonine	dicyclomine
Dymelor	Demerol
Dymelor	Pamelor
Dyrenium	Pyridium
Ecotrin	Akineton
Ecotrin	Edecrin
Edecrin	Ecotrin
Elavil	Aldoril
Elavil	Equanil
Elavil	Mellaril
Empirin	Enduron
encainide	flecainide
Endep	Depen
Enduron	Empirin
Enduron	Imuran
Enduronyl	Inderal

enflurane	isoflurane
Enkaid	Cankaid
Equanil	Elavil
Ery-Tab	Eryc
Eryc	Ery-Tab
Esidrix	Lasix
Esimil	Estinyl
Esimil	Ismelin
Estinyl	Esimil
Estratab	Ethatab
Ethamolin	ethanol
ethanol	Ethamolin
Ethatab	Estratab
etidocaine	etidronate
etidronate	etidocaine
etidronate	etretinate
etretinate	etidronate
Eurax	Serax
Eurax	Urex
Excedrin	Dexedrine
Factrel	Sectral
Feldene	Seldane
fenoprofen	flurbiprofen
fentanyl	alfentanil
Feosol	Feostat
Feosol	Fer-in-Sol
Feosol	Festal
Feosol	Fluosol
Feostat	Feosol
Fer-in-Sol	Feosol
Festal	Feosol
Festal	Festalan
Festalan	Festal
Fiogesic	Wygesic
Fiorinal	Florinef
Flaxedil	Flexeril
flecainide	encainide
Flexeril	Flaxedil
Flexeril	Floxin
Florinef	Fiorinal
Floxin	Flexeril
flunisolide	fluocinonide
fluocinolone	fluocinonide
fluocinonide	flunisolide
fluocinonide	fluocinolone

Fluosol	Feosol
flurbiprofen	fenoprofen
folic acid	folinic acid
folinic acid	folic acid
fosinopril	lisinopril
Fostex	pHisoHex
Fulvicin	Furacin
Furacin	Fulvicin
Gamastan	Garamycin
Gantanol	Gantrisin
Gantrisin	Gantanol
Garamycin	Gamastan
Garamycin	kanamycin
Garamycin	Terramycin
Gelfoam	Ger-O-Foam
gentamicin	kanamycin
Ger-O-Foam	Gelfoam
Glaucon	glucagon
glipizide	glyburide
glucagon	Glaucon
glutethimide	guanethidine
glyburide	glipizide
guanethidine	glutethimide
Halcion	Healon
Haldol	Halog
Halog	Haldol
Halotestin	halothane
halothane	Halotestin
Healon	Halcion
Hespan	Histaspan
Hexadrol	Hexalol
Hexalol	Hexadrol
Histaspan	Hespan
Hycodan	Vicodin
Hycomine	Vicodin
hydralazine	hydrochlorothiazide
hydralazine	hydroxyzine
hydrochlorothiazide	hydralazine
hydrochlorothiazide	hydroflumethiazide
hydrocortisone	hydroxychloroquine
hydroflumethiazide	hydrochlorothiazide
Hydropres	Diupres
hydroxychloroquine	hydrocortisone
hydroxyurea	hydroxyzine
hydroxyzine	hydralazine

hydroxyzine	hydroxyurea
Hygroton	Regroton
Hyper-Tet	HyperHep
Hyper-Tet	Hyperstat
HyperHep	Hyper-Tet
HyperHep	Hyperstat
Hyperstat	Hyper-Tet
Hyperstat	HyperHep
Hyperstat	Nitrostat
Hytone	Vytone
Idamycin	Adriamycin
Idamycin	Iodo-Niacin
Iletin	Lente
Imferon	Intropin
Imferon	imipramine
Imferon	Imuran
imipramine	desipramine
imipramine	Imferon
imipramine	norpramin
Imuran	Enduron
Imuran	Imferon
Imuran	Inderal
Inderal	Enduronyl
Inderal	Imuran
Inderal	Inderide
Inderal	Isordil
Inderide	Inderal
Indocin	Lincocin
Indocin	Minocin
Inocor	Norcuron
Intropin	Ditropan
Intropin	Imferon
Intropin	Isoptin
iodine	Iopidine
iodine	Lodine
Iodo-Niacin	Idamycin
Ionamin	Tenormin
Iopidine	iodine
Iopidine	Lodine
Ismelin	Esimil
Ismelin	Isuprel
Ismelin	Ritalin
isoflurane	enflurane
Isoptin	Intropin
Isopto Carpine	Isopto Eserine

Isopto Eserine	Isopto Carpine
Isordil	Inderal
Isordil	Isuprel
Isuprel	Ismelin
Isuprel	Isordil
K-Lor	Kaochlor
K-Lor	Klor-Con
K-Phos Neutral	Neutra-Phos-K
kanamycin	Garamycin
kanamycin	gentamicin
Kaochlor	K-Lor
kaolin	Kaon
Kaon	kaolin
Keflex	Keflin
Keflin	Keflex
Kemadrin	Coumadin
Kenalog	Ketalar
Ketalar	Kenalog
Klonopin	clonidine
Klor-Con	K-Lor
Klotrix	Liotrix
Lanoxin	Levoxine
Lanoxin	Levsinex
Larotid	Lomotil
Lasan	Lasix
Lasix	Esidrix
Lasix	Lasan
Lasix	Lidex
Lente	Iletin
Leukeran	Leukine
Leukine	Leukeran
Levodopa	methyldopa
Levoxine	Lanoxin
Levisinex	Lanoxin
Lidex	Cidex
Lidex	Lasix
Lincocin	Cleocin
Lincocin	Indocin
Lincocin	Minocin
Lioresal	lisinopril
Liotrix	Klotrix
lisinopril	fosinopril
lisinopril	Lioresal
lobeline	Lodine
Lodine	codeine

Lodine	iodine
Lodine	Iopidine
Lodine	lobeline
Lomotil	Larotid
Lopressor	Lopurin
Lopurin	Lopressor
Lopurin	Lupron
lorazepam	alprazolam
lorazepam	temazepam
Lotrimin	Otrivin
Luminal	Tuinal
Lupron	Lopurin
Lupron	Nuprin
Maalox	Marax
Mandol	Nadolol
Marax	Maalox
Matulane	Modane
Maxidex	Maxzide
Maxzide	Maxidex
mazindol	mebendazole
Mebaral	Mellaril
Mebaral	Tegretol
mebendazole	mazindol
Mellaril	Elavil
Mellaril	Mebaral
Mellaril	Moderil
melphalan	mephyton
meperidine	meprobamate
Mephyton	malphalan
meprivacaine	bupivacaine
meprobamate	meperidine
Meprospan	Naprosyn
methyldopa	Levodopa
metolazone	minoxidil
metryapone	metyrosine
metryosine	metyrapone
Mexitil	Mezlin
Mezlin	Azlin
Mezlin	Mexitil
miconazole	Micronase
miconazole	Micronor
Micronase	miconazole
Micronor	miconazole
Midrin	Mydfrin
Milontin	Miltown

Milontin	Mylanta
Miltown	Milontin
Minocin	Indocin
Minocin	Lincocin
Minocin	Mithracin
Minocin	niacin
minoxidil	metolazone
Mithracin	Minocin
mithramycin	mitomycin
mitomycin	mitotane
mitotane	mitomycin
Modane	Matulane
Modane	Mudrane
Moderil	Mellaril
Modicon	Mylicon
monopril	ramipril
Mudrane	Modane
Myambutol	Nembutal
Mycelex	Myoflex
Myciguent	Mycitracin
Mycitracin	Myciguent
Mydfrin	Midrin
Mylanta	Milontin
Myleran	Mylicon
Mylicon	Modicon
Mylicon	Myleran
Myochrysine	vincristine
Myoflex	Mycelex
Nadolol	Mandol
Naldecon	Nalfon
Nalfon	Naldecon
naloxone	naltrexone
naltrexone	naloxone
Naprosyn	Meprospan
Naprosyn	Nebcin
Navane	Nubain
Nebcin	Naprosyn
Nembutal	Myambutol
Neutra-Phos-K	K-Phos Neutral
niacin	Minocin
Nicobin	Nitro-Bid
Nicorette	Nordette
Nilstat	Nitrostat
Nilstat	Nystatin
Nitro-Bid	Nicobin

nitroglycerin	Nitroglyn
Nitroglyn	nitroglycerin
Nitrostat	Hyperstat
Nitrostat	Nilstat
Nitrostat	Nystatin
Norcuron	Inocor
Nordette	Nicorette
Norgesic Forte	Norgesic 40
Norgesic 40	Norgesic Forte
Norlutate	Norlutin
Norlutin	Norlutate
Norpace	norpramin
norpramin	imipramine
norpramin	Norpace
norpramin	nortriptyline
norpramin	Tenormin
nortriptyline	norpramin
Nubain	Navane
Nuprin	Lupron
Nydrazid	nylidrin
nylidrin	Nydrazid
Nystatin	Nilstat
Nystatin	Nitrostat
Omnipaque	Amipaque
Ophthaine	Ophthetic
Ophthetic	Ophthaine
Ophthochlor	Ophthocort
Opthocort	Ophthochlor
Optimine	Optimyd
Optimyd	Optimine
Oracin	Orasone
Orasone	Oracin
Oretic	Oreton
Oreton	Oretic
Orexin	Ornex
Orinase	Ornade
Orinase	Ornex
Ornade	Orinase
Ornade	Ornex
Ornex	Orexin
Ornex	Orinase
Ornex	Ornade
Otrivin	Lotrimin
Pamelor	Dymelor
Pamine	Pelamine

Panadol	pindolol
Panadol	Valadol
Panadol	Panafil
Panafil	Panadol
Pantopon	Parafon
Pantopon	Protopam
Parafon	Pantopon
paregoric	Percogesic
Pathilon	Pathocil
Pathocil	Bactocill
Pathocil	Pathilon
Pathocil	Placidyl
Pavabid	Pavatine
Pavatine	Pavabid
Pediapred	PediaProfen
PediaProfen	Pediapred
Pelamine	Pamine
Pelamine	pemoline
pemoline	Pelamine
penicillamine	penicillin
penicillin	penicillamine
penicillin	Polycillin
pentobarbital	phenobarbital
Pentrax	Permax
Percodan	Decadron
Percodan	Percogesic
Percodan	Periactin
Percogesic	paregoric
Percogesic	Percodan
Periactin	Percodan
Permax	Pentrax
Phenaphen	Phenergan
phenelzine	Phenylzin
Phenergan	Phenaphen
phenobarbital	pentobarbital
phentermine	phentolamine
phentolamine	phentermine
Phenylzin	phenelzine
pHisoHex	Fostex
pHisoHex	Phos-Ex
Phos-Ex	pHisoHex
PhosChol	PhosLo
PhosChol	Phosphocol
PhosLo	PhosChol
Phosphocol	PhosChol

Phrenilin	Trinalin
pindolol	Panadol
Pitocin	Pitressin
Petressin	Pitocin
Placidyl	Pathocil
Polycillin	penicillin
Ponstel	Pronestyl
pralidoxime	Pramoxine
pralidoxime	pyridoxine
Pramoxine	pralidoxime
prazepam	prazosin
prozosin	prazepam
prazosin	prednisone
prednisolone	prednisone
prednisone	prazosin
prednisone	prednisolone
Priscoline	Apresoline
procaine	Procan
procaine	Prokine
Procan	procaine
Prokine	procaine
Proloprim	Protropin
promazine	promethazine
promethazine	chlorpromazine
promethazine	promazine
Pronestyl	Ponstel
Pronestyl	Prostaphlin
proparacaine	propoxyphene
propoxyphene	proparacaine
Prostaphlin	Pronestyl
protamine	Protpam
protamine	Protropin
Protopam	Pantopon
Protopam	protamine
Protopam	Protropin
Protropin	Proloprim
Protropin	protamine
Protropin	Protopam
Pyridium	Dyrenium
Pyridium	pyridoxine
pyridoxine	pralidoxime
pyridoxine	Pyridium
Quarzan	Questran
Questran	Quarzan
Quinamm	quinidine

quinidine	clonidine
quinidine	Quinamm
quinidine	quinine
quinidine	Quinora
quinine	quinidine
Quinora	quinidine
ramipril	monopril
Regroton	Hygroton
Restoril	Vistaril
Ribavirin	riboflavin
riboflavin	Ribavirin
Rifadin	Ritalin
Ritalin	Ismelin
Ritalin	Rifadin
salsalate	sucralfate
salsalate	sulfasalazine
Sandimmune	Sandostatin
Sandostatin	Sandimmune
Sebulex	Sebutone
Sebutone	Sebulex
Sectral	Factrel
Sectral	Septra
Seldane	Feldene
Septa	Septra
Septra	Ceptaz
Septra	Sectral
Septra	Septa
Serax	Eurax
Serax	Xerac
Serentil	Surital
simethicone	cimetidine
Slow FE	Slow-K
Slow-K	Slow FE
somatrem	somatropin
somatropin	somatrem
Stilphostrol	Disophrol
sucralfate	salsalate
sufentanil	alfentanil
sulfamethizole	sulfamethoxazole
sulfamethoxazole	sulfamethizole
sulfasalazine	salsalate
Surbex	Surfak
Surfak	Surbex
Surital	Serentil
Sustacal	Sustaire

Sustaire	Sustacal
Tagamet	Tegopen
Talacen	Taractan
Talacen	Tinactin
Taractan	Talacen
Taractan	Tinactin
Tedral	Teldrin
Tedral	Tridil
Tegopen	Tagamet
Tegopen	Tegretol
Tegopen	Tegrin
Tegretol	Mebaral
Tegretol	Tegopen
Tegretol	Tegrin
Tegrin	Tegopen
Tegrin	Tegretol
Teldrin	Tedral
Temaril	Demerol
Temaril	Tepanil
temazepam	lorazepam
Ten-K	Tenex
Tenex	Ten-K
Tenex	Xanax
Tenormin	Ionamin
Tenormin	norpramin
Tepanil	Temaril
Tepanil	Tofranil
terconazole	tioconazole
Terramycin	Garamycin
testolactone	testosterone
testosterone	testolactone
Theolair	Thyrolar
Thiacide	Dyazide
thiamine	Thorazine
Thorazine	thiamine
Thyrar	Thyrolar
Thyrolar	Theolair
Thyrolar	Thyrar
Ticar	Tigan
Tigan	Ticar
timolol	atenolol
Timoptic	Viroptic
Tinactin	Talacen
Tinactin	Taractan
Tindal	Trental

tioconazole	terconazole
tobramycin	Tobricin
Tobricin	tobramycin
Tofranil	Tepanil
tolazamide	tolbutamide
tolbutamide	tolazamide
Trandate HCl	Trandate HCT
Trandate HCT	Trandate HCl
Trandate	Trendar
Trandate	Trental
Trendar	Trandate
Trendar	Trental
Trental	Tindal
Trental	Trandate
Trental	Trendar
tretinoin	trientine
triamcinolone	Triaminicol
Triaminic	Triaminicin
Triaminic	TriHemic
Traminicin	Triaminic
Triaminicol	triamcinolone
triamterene	trimipramine
trichloacetic acid	dichloracetic acid
Tridil	Tedral
trientine	tretinoin
TriHemic	Triaminic
trimeprazine	trimipramine
trimipramine	triamterene
trimipramine	trimeprazine
Trimox	Diamox
Trimox	Tylox
Trinalin	Phrenilin
Tronolane	Tronothane
Tronothane	Tronolane
Tuinal	Luminal
Tuinal	Tylenol
Tylenol	Tuinal
Tylox	Trimox
Tylox	Wymox
Urex	Eurax
V-Cillin	Bicillin
V-Cillin	Wycillin
Valadol	Panadol
Valium	Valpin
Valpin	Valium

Vanceril	Vansil
Vansil	Vanceril
Vasocidin	Vasodilan
Vasodilan	Vasocidin
Vasosulf	Velosef
Velosef	Vasosulf
Ventolin	Benylin
VePesid	Versed
Verelan	Vivarin
Versed	VePesid
Vicodin	Hycodan
Vicodin	Hycomine
vincristine	Myochrysine
Viroptic	Timoptic
Visine	Visken
Visken	Visine
Vistaril	Restoril
Vivarin	Verelan
Vontrol	Bontril
Vytone	Hytone
Wycillin	V-Cillin
Wygesic	Fiogesic
Wymox	Tylox
Xanax	Tenex
Xanax	Zantac
Xerac	Serax
Zantac	Xanax
Zarontin	Zaroxolyn
Zarontin	Zentron
Zaroxolyn	Zarontin
Zentron	Zarontin
Zestril	Desyrel
Zestril	Zostrix
ZORprin	Zyloprim
Zostrix	Zestril
Zyloprim	ZORprin

Glossary

absorption: The process that enables the drug to be distributed into the bloodstream.

acetylcholine: A neurotransmitter that plays an important role in transmitting nerve impulses. Its action is blocked by anticholinergic drugs.

addiction: Physical and/or psychological dependence on a substance.

adrenergic: An agent that produces stimulating adrenalin-like effects on the sympathetic nervous system.

adverse effect: A symptom that occurs when a side effect becomes severe.

allergen: A substance capable of causing an allergy or allergic reaction.

allergic reaction: A hypersensitivity to medications.

allergy: An antibody-antigen allergen reaction; hypersensitivity to a substance.

amphetamine: A stimulant to the central nervous system.

ampules: Small, sterile, prefilled glass containers usually designed for one-time usage.

analgesic: A drug given to relieve pain without loss of consciousness.

analog (analogue): A substance structurally or chemically similar to another related drug or chemical for the purpose of changing the original drug's characteristics to produce an improved drug with fewer side effects or more therapeutic action.

anaphylaxis: An allergic hypersensitivity usually to a protein substance or drug; a severe, life-threatening allergic reaction accompanied by vasodilation, lowered blood pressure, and shock.

antagonist: A drug that opposes a bodily system or expected effect.

anesthetic: A drug that causes loss of sensation and insensibility to pain or touch.

antacid: A drug that neutralizes acidity, especially in the digestive tract.

antagonist: Undesirable effect which can produce an unfavorable response by heightening side effects when two drugs interact.

antianaphylactic: Prevention of anaphylaxis. Often attained by administering repeated doses of a sensitizing substance too small to call an anaphylactic reaction; a way of desensitizing.

antianginal: A drug that relieves chest pain.

antianxiety drugs: Drugs used to relieve anxiety and emotional tension.

antiarrhythmic: A drug that prevents cardiac arrhythmias.

antibiotic: A drug used to kill living microorganisms, including gram-positive and gram-negative bacteria, that cause infection.

antibody: A protein substance which develops in response to and reacts with an invading antigen.

anticoagulant: A drug used to prevent blood clotting.

anticonvulsant: A drug that relieves or prevents convulsions.

antidiabetic: A drug that prevents or relieves diabetes.

antidiarrheal: A drug that relieves or corrects diarrhea.

antidote: Any substance that neutralizes or counteracts the effects of a poison.

antiemetic: A drug that prevents or relieves vomiting.

antifungal: A synthetic drug that destroys or inhibits fungal growth and yeast infections.

antigen: A foreign substance (virus, bacterium, or toxin) that induces the production of antibodies.

antihistamine: A drug used to treat and relieve allergy symptoms (such as hay fever), and relieves symptoms of the common cold, urticaria, and pruritus.

anti-inflammatory: A drug used to treat and relieve pain, swelling, and tenderness.

antinauseant: A drug used to prevent or decrease nausea.

antipruritic: A drug, ointment, or solution that relieves itching.

antipsychotic: A drug used to treat schizophrenia, paranoia, and other psychotic disorders.

antipyretic: A drug given to reduce fever.

antiseptic: A topical drug used on living tissue which prevents or inhibits the growth of microorganisms, especially bacteria (it does not necessarily kill them).

antispasmodic: A drug used to relieve or prevent muscular contractions, spasms, and convulsions.

antitussive: A drug given to relieve a cough.

antiviral: A drug used to combat viral infections and diseases.

APhA: American Pharmaceutical Association.

aphrodisiac: A drug used to arouse or increase sexual desire.

apothecary system: System used by pharmacists in preparing prescriptions; consists of roman numerals and common fractions.

astringent: A substance that produces shrinkage of mucous membranes or other tissues and decreases secretion.

average dose: The amount of medication taken to produce effective results with a minimal toxic effect.

bactericide: A substance that kills bacteria.

bacteriostatic: A substance that inhibits the growth of bacteria.

bolus: A single dose of a drug that can be injected into an existing IV line through a rubber stopper (port).

bore (synonymous with gauge): The inside diameter of a needle. Unlike the gauge, the bore is never assigned a specific number but is designated small or large.

brand name: See *trade name.*

buccal administration: The method by which a medication is held between the gum and cheek.

buffered analgesic: A pill containing an antacid to reduce acidity.

butterfly needle: A specially designed needle of short length and high gauge. It has color-coded plastic tabs on each side to facilitate control of the needle during insertion. They are often used to start IVs on premature babies and geriatric patients with poor veins.

cancer: A tumor or unnatural growth in the body.

Candida: A genus of yeast-like fungi.

carcinogen: An agent that produces cancer.

carminative: An agent used to expel gas from the GI tract.

catalyst: A substance that increases the speed of a chemical reaction but is not used up nor permanently changed in any way by the reaction.

cathartic: A drug used to increase and hasten evacuation of the bowel (a laxative).

CD: An abbreviation for "continual dosing," usually part of the trade name (Cardizem CD).

chemical name: Drug name determined by its precise chemical description and molecular structure.

chemotherapy: The use of chemical agents to treat or control a disease. It is used when cancer is disseminated, when it cannot be surgically removed, or when it fails to respond to radiation.

cholinergic: A type of receptor activated by the neurotransmitter acetylcholine.

cocaine: A CNS (central nervous system) stimulant extracted from leaves of the Erythroxylan coca plant. It is a Schedule II drug used as a surface anesthesia of the ear, nose, throat, rectum, and vagina. Street names include blow, coke, flake, gold dust, rock, snow, and white girl. Cocaine combined with heroin is known as a speed ball.

contraindication: A symptom indicating inappropriateness of a drug or treatment. A specific factor physicians consider prior to selecting medication for an individual.

Controlled Substance Act (CSA): Act requiring all medical practitioners who will have an occasion to dispense, prescribe, or administer a controlled substance to have a narcotic license granted by the DEA.

controlled substances: Substances or medications that have the potential for addiction and abuse if taken without close supervision by a physician.

corticosteroid: A hormone produced by adrenal glands, or a topical or oral drug used to reduce inflammation and treat allergic rhinitis.

CR: An abbreviation for "controlled release," usually part of the trade name (Norpace CR).

cream: A semisolid (emulsion—a mixture of two liquids not mutually soluble) of fat globules in a water base.

DEA: See *Drug Enforcement Administration.*

decongestant: A drug used to symptomatically treat nasal congestion; constricts dilated arterioles reducing nasal blood flow and improving drainage.

dependence: A severe attachment to a drug or agent; an addiction.

depressant: Any agent or drug that reduces the function or activity of a body system such as a sedative or anesthetic.

depression: An unnatural state of lethargy, inactivity, and sadness.

desensitize: To lessen the sensitivity by administering an antigen.

diaphoretic: A drug used to induce and increase perspiration.

disinfectant (germicide): A chemical used on inanimate objects that kill or inhibit growth of microorganisms. It is used to sterilize instruments, but not used on the human body.

diuretic: A drug used to increase the excretion of urine; used to treat edema and hypertension.

dosage: The amount of medication to be administered.

dose: A specified amount of medicinal preparation to be administered at one time.

drug: Any chemical substance that affects body function.

drug abuse: The harmful, nonmedical use of a mind-altering drug.

drug of choice: A drug shown to be of particular clinical value in treating a specific diseased state. It is preferred above all other similar drugs because of its superior therapeutic results.

Drug Enforcement Administration: Administration established to regulate the manufacturing and dispensing of dangerous and potentially abused drugs.

drug tolerance: A decreased susceptibility to the effects of a drug caused by continued use.

DS: An abbreviation for a double dosage (double-strength); usually part of the trade name (Bactrim DS).

emetic: A drug that stimulates vomiting.

emollient: A substance that softens the skin and soothes irritation.

emulsions: Fine droplets of either oil in water or water in oil. They must be vigorously shaken to ensure mixing prior to use.

enteric coating: This special coating allows pills to pass through the stomach and dissolve in the small intestine. This type of coating is used to minimize stomach irritation, but it also takes longer to absorb.

enzyme: A substance formed by living cells that promotes a particular chemical reaction in the body by functioning as a catalyst.

exacerbation: When the symptoms of a disease are most severe.

excretion: The process of eliminating the drug from the body.

expectorant: A drug used to liquify mucus from the respiratory tract which increases secretions, making it easier to expel mucus.

extended release: Slow dissolving; prolongs release of agent into the system.

FDA: Food and Drug Administration.

gauge: The inside diameter of a needle. The smaller the number, the larger the diameter.

general anesthesia: The introduction of an agent that eliminates pain and voluntary muscle control, then induces unconsciousness.

generic name: Drug name given before the drug becomes official.

habit forming: The condition whereby drugs are routinely taken as a matter of course, not as a matter of necessity. Withdrawal symptoms are not seen on cessation of the habit. User becomes accustomed to frequent use.

habituation: Becoming accustomed to taking a drug (a psychological dependence).

half-life: The time required for drug levels in the serum to decrease from 100 percent to 50 percent. The half-life of a drug can be significantly prolonged with liver or kidney disease. For example, digoxin (Lanoxin) has a half-life of approximately 30 hours. Geriatric patients with poor liver and kidney functioning often develop levels of toxicity because circulating levels of the active drug remain high for long periods of time.

hematinic: An agent that tends to increase the hemoglobin content of the blood; usually contains iron.

histamine: An amino acid that produces the symptoms of allergic reactions.

hormone: An agent secreted by the endocrine glands that produces or alters bodily functions.

hypersensitivity: Excessive or abnormal sensitivity/susceptibility to the action of a given agent.

hypnotic: A drug used to produce sleep.

immunization: A process of inducing or providing immunity by administering an artificial immunizing agent. It is usually given in childhood to reduce the occurrence of vaccine-preventable diseases.

immunosuppressive: An agent that interferes with the body systems that resist infection and foreign materials.

infection: The process of a pathogenic agent invading the body, multiplying, and causing injury.

inhalation: The act of drawing air into the lungs by breathing; medication administration by means of a special apparatus such as an inhalator, vaporizer, atomizer, nebulizer, intermittent positive pressure machine, or respirator.

initial dose: The first dose administered.

injection: The act of forcing liquid into a body part; medication is administered either directly into the bloodstream or tissue.

instillation: Application of a drug into body cavities such as the conjunctival sacs of the eyes, ears, nose, throat, vagina, and rectum.

insulin syringe: A special syringe designed to measure only insulin. It is calibrated in units; all other syringes are calibrated in milliliters.

intrinsic factor: A substance in the gastric wall that is necessary for vitamin B12 absorption.

irrigation: The cleansing of a canal by flushing with water or other fluids; used in the washing of a wound.

IV drip: Drug is mixed with a fluid in a bottle or bag that is administered continuously over several hours.

IV push: Drug is virtually pushed into the IV line.

JCAHD: Joint Commission on Accreditation of Healthcare Organizations.

L-dopa: L is the abbreviation for levorotary, a term used to describe a drug's molecules which are arranged in a way that bends polarized light to the left.

LA: An abbreviation for long-acting. It is usually part of the trade name of sustained-release, long-acting drugs such as Entex LA.

laxative: A mild cathartic that loosens and promotes bowel movements without discomfort.

lethal dose: The amount of a drug that will cause death.

liquid preparations: Preparations that contain drugs that are dissolved or suspended, and when taken internally (with the exception of emulsions), are rapidly absorbed through the stomach or intestinal wall.

loading dose: An amount that is generally twice the maintenance dose; given if the therapeutic effect of a drug is desired immediately to treat a medical crisis. This promptly raises the serum levels of the drug to the therapeutic range to initiate treatment. The loading dose is given only once, then maintenance doses are used for subsequent treatment.

local anesthesia: Introduction of a drug, usually injected, that temporarily eliminates pain by interfering with local nerve transmission, causing a deadening in a small, limited area.

local effect: Effect limited to the immediate area where the medicine is applied.

long-acting: See *LA*.

LSD: Lysergic acid diethylamide. Taken orally, it is frequently absorbed in a sugar cube. LSD is a Schedule I drug. Its street name is usually "acid."

maintenance dose: The standard dose prescribed by the physician. It is generally one-half the loading dose.

marijuana: The dried, flowering tops and leaves (and occasionally seeds and stems) of the Cannabis sativa plant. It is often hand-rolled into cigarettes and smoked; a Schedule I drug. (A synthetic variation has been approved as an antiemetic for cancer treatment.) Street names include Acapulco gold, grass, joint, Mary Jane, pot, and reefer.

maximal dose: The largest amount of drug given, still producing the desired effect.

medicine: The science and art of healing; seeks to save lives and relieve suffering.

metabolism: The chemical energy of foodstuffs transformed to mechanical energy or heat.

metastasis: The spread of cancer cells from one body part to another.

microorganism: An organism not visible to the naked eye that may or may not produce a disease.

minerals: Naturally occurring, inorganic substances necessary to body function.

minimal dose: See *therapeutic dose*.

miotic: A drug that causes the pupil to contract.

mydriatic: A drug that causes the pupil to dilate.

narcotic: A drug used to relieve pain and produce sleep or stupor.

needles: Slender, hollow instruments which are classified according to gauge and length and are used to inject liquids.

New Drugs List: Annual publication by the Council on Pharmacy of the AMA.

NSAIDs: Nonsteroidal anti-inflammatory drugs.

ointment: (Abbreviation: ung) A semisolid, medicated emulsion of water globules in a fat base for external topical application.

oral: Medication given by mouth.

OTC: See *over-the-counter*.

over-the-counter: Drugs or medications taken not requiring a physician's order.

oxytocic: A drug used to produce uterine contractions.

palliative: A drug which provides relief of symptoms but does not cure the disease.

parenteral: All methods of giving medications by means of a needle or cannula introduced through the skin, including sub-Q, IM, IV, intraspinal, intrasternal, intracapsular, and intraorbital.

pathogen: A microorganism capable of causing disease (virus, bacterium, or fungus).

PCP: Phencyclidene. It may come in a powder, tablet, or capsule form, or it can also be injected. Schedule I drug; no legal use in the United States. Street names include angel dust, cosmos, jet, peace pill, super joint, and whack.

PDR: Physicians' Desk Reference, the most widely used drug reference book.

peak levels: Measurements which indicate the highest serum level achieved following a single dose of a drug. They are used to determine if serum levels of a drug are high enough to produce a therapeutic effect or are too high, which would cause toxicity. Peak levels are determined by blood tests.

pharmacist: Qualified professional who prepares drugs and prescriptions.

pharmacodynamics: The study of drugs and their actions on the body.

pharmacokinetics: The study of the metabolism and action of drugs within the body with particular emphasis on the time required for absorption, duration, distribution, and method of excretion.

pharmacology: The science that deals with the study of chemical substances and their effect on living organisms. It is one of the oldest branches of medicine.

pharmacotherapeutics: Studies the relationship between drugs and the treatment of diseases.

pharmacy: Facility where drugs are legally prepared, compounded, and dispensed.

piggyback: When a drug is mixed in a very small bag or bottle, and it is connected to a port and administered into the existing IV line to empty within an hour.

placebo: An inactive preparation commonly known as sugar pills. They are in controlled pharmaceutical studies to determine effectiveness of a tested medication. In most situations, the patient is unaware he or she is being administered a placebo. It may be given in place of an actual drug to gratify the patient.

prophylactic: A drug used to prevent the development of a disease; includes vaccines, birth control pills, hormones, or vitamins.

proprietary name: See *trade name.*

prostaglandins: Short-acting hormones that perform many functions in the body and exert their effect close to the site of production.

prothrombin: A protein produced by the liver necessary for normal blood coagulation.

prothrombin time: A measurement of the prothrombin level in the blood. This measurement is performed routinely to assess the effectiveness of anticoagulant therapy.

SA: An abbreviation for sustained action. It is usually part of the trade name of sustained release, long-acting drugs, such as Choledyl SA.

sedative: A drug that exerts a quiet, relaxing effect; relieves anxiety without inducing sleep.

semisolid preparations: Include suppositories, ointments, and creams.

shock: A sudden drop in blood pressure due to injury or blood loss.

side effect: Any action or effect other than the desired effect.

signa: Latin for "label."

SL: An abbreviation for sublingual. It is usually part of the trade name, such as Isordil SL.

solid preparations: Tablets, capsules, caplets, and lozenges. (Occasionally powders are included as a fifth type of solid preparation as seen in chapter 5.)

solutions (sol): One or more substances completely dissolved.

Spansules: A registered trademark of SmithKline pharmaceutical company, designating a slow-release capsule such as Compazine Spansules.

SR: An abbreviation for slow release or sustained release. It is usually part of the trade name, such as Theospan SR.

steroid: A compound which accelerates physical development by increasing body weight and muscular strength. It may be taken orally or injected directly into muscle. Street names include roids, juice, and d-ball.

stimulant: A drug that temporarily increases activity or hastens actions in the body or in an organ; counteracts depression.

subscription: Specific directions for the pharmacist such as route of administration, total number of tablets or capsules to dispense, dosage and frequency, length of treatment, and/or the number of refills permitted.

suppositories: (Abbreviation: supp) A semisolid base of soap, glycerinated gelatin, or cocoa butter containing a drug for introduction into the rectum, vagina, or urethra, where it dissolves when subject to body heat.

sustained action: See *SA*.

sustained (slow) release: See *SR*.

synergists: Drugs which react favorably together. One drug can favorably enhance the effect of another drug.

systemic effect: Effect felt throughout the patient's body.

therapeutic dose: The smallest amount of drug that will produce a desired effect.

therapeutic effect: The desired effect; that which will treat or cure the medical condition.

therapeutic index: A measurement calculated during animal testing of any new drug. It reflects the relative margin of safety inherent between the dose needed to produce a therapeutic effect and the dose which produces toxic effects. The higher the therapeutic index the better, as it indicates the drug has a wide margin of safety. Penicillin has a therapeutic index of greater than 100. The therapeutic index of digoxin is less than 2. It is not uncommon for patients taking a therapeutic dose of digoxin to begin to exhibit symptoms of toxicity.

time release: See *extended release.*

titrate: The smallest dosage that will produce the desired effect for a specific individual.

tolerance: The capacity for enduring a large amount of a substance without exhibiting any adverse effects.

topical: Substances applied to the skin such as unguents, ointments, creams, sprays, emulsions, powders, liniments, or liquids.

toxic dose: Any dosage that causes a poisonous or potentially dangerous situation for the patient.

toxic effect: When the serum level of a drug rises beyond the therapeutic level to a level of toxicity.

toxicology: The study of poisons.

toxin: The poisonous substance released by microorganisms.

trade name: Specific drug name indicating FDA has given final marketing approval; selected by manufacturer.

tranquilizer: A drug used to reduce anxiety without clouding consciousness; a sedative.

transdermal: Medication delivered through the skin by means of a patch.

trough levels: A measurement determined by a blood test indicating the lowest serum level of a drug which occurs just before the next dose is to be given.

unit dosage: Medications that are premeasured and individually packaged in a per-dose basis.

vasopressor: A drug that produces vasoconstriction and an increase in blood pressure.

vial: A small glass bottle with a rubber stopper containing a liquid or powder for injection. The rubber stopper allows repeated doses of the drug to be withdrawn from the same vial.

withdrawal: Cessation of administration of a drug, especially a narcotic, to which a patient has become physically or psychologically addicted.

Index

P

Painkillers
    narcotic, 136
    nonnarcotic, 121, 134, 135
Palliative, defined, 78
Parenteral, defined, 79
Parenteral administration, 53–63
Pathogen, defined, 79
Patient information sheet, illustrated, 64, 65
Patient responsibility for taking medication correctly, 63–65
PCP, defined, 79
PDR, *see* Physician's Desk Reference
Peak levels, defined, 79
Pharmacist, 3; defined, 11
Pharmacodynamics, defined, 2
Pharmacokinetics, defined, 2
Pharmacology
    changes in, 4–5
    defined, 2
    historical progression, 2
Pharmacotherapeutics, defined, 2
Pharmacy, defined, 11
Phrophylactic, defined, 35
Physician's Desk Reference (PDR), 113
    additional information in, 114–15
    additional reference materials, 118
    defined, 79
    sections of, 114
    steps for using, 115–18
    supplements, 113
Piggyback, defined, 61
Placebo, defined, 79
Prescribing professions, 11
Prescription abbreviations, common, 81–82
Prescription labels, 106–7
Prescription medications versus over-the-counter drugs, 105
Prescription slip content, 105–6
Prescriptions
    clerical steps in refilling, 109
    refilling, 108–9

Prophylactic, defined, 79
Prophylaxis, 35
Proprietary (trade) name, defined, 17
Prostaglandins, defined, 79
Prothrombin, defined, 79
Prothrombin time, defined, 79

R

Respirator, illustrated, 51
Roman numerals, 88–89
Routes of administration, 44–63

S

SA, defined, 79
Schedule of narcotics, 13; illustrated, 15
Sedative, defined, 79
Semisolid preparations, 24–26; defined, 24
Shock, defined, 79
Side effects, defined, 39, 79
SL, defined, 79
Solid preparations, 23–24; defined, 23
Solute, defined, 26
Solutions, 26–28
Solvent, defined, 26
Spansules, 23; defined, 79
Spinal block, 68
Spray, 28
SR, defined, 79
Standard syringe, 54
Steroids, defined, 79
Stimulant, defined, 80
Subcutaneous injections, 57
Sublingual administration, 47–48
Subscription, defined, 106
Superstition versus modern medicine, 3
Suppositories, defined, 24
Suspension, 26
Sustained action, defined, 80
Sustained (slow) release, defined, 80
Symbols, commonly used, 154
Synergists, defined, 35